ESOPHAGEAL CANCER AND BEYOND

Edited by **Jianyuan Chai**

Esophageal Cancer and Beyond

http://dx.doi.org/10.5772/intechopen.73883
Edited by Jianyuan Chai

Contributors

Jacqueline Oxenberg, Emanuele Salvatore Aragona, Jianyuan Chai, Ljiljana Širić, Marinela Rosso, Yi Zhang, Tian Wang

Notice

Statements and opinions expressed in the chapters are these of the individual contributors and not necessarily those of the editors or publisher. No responsibility is accepted for the accuracy of information contained in the published chapters. The publisher assumes no responsibility for any damage or injury to persons or property arising out of the use of any materials, instructions, methods or ideas contained in the book.

First published in London, United Kingdom, 2018 by IntechOpen
IntechOpen is the global imprint of INTECHOPEN LIMITED, registered in England and Wales, registration number: 11086078, The Shard, 25th floor, 32 London Bridge Street
London, SE19SG – United Kingdom
Printed in Croatia

British Library Cataloguing-in-Publication Data
A catalogue record for this book is available from the British Library

Additional hard copies can be obtained from orders@intechopen.com

Esophageal Cancer and Beyond , Edited by Jianyuan Chai
p. cm.
Print ISBN 978-1-78984-412-2
Online ISBN 978-1-78984-413-9

For EU product safety concerns:
IN TECH d.o.o., Prolaz Marije Krucifikse Kozulić 3, 51000 Rijeka, Croatia,
info@intechopen.com or visit our website at intechopen.com.

Meet the editor

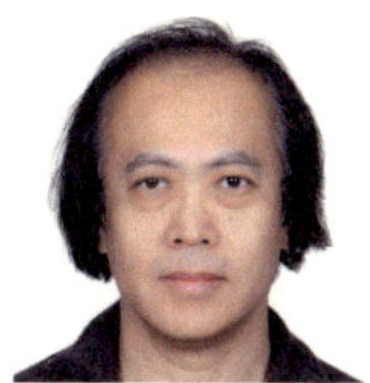

Dr. Chai received his Ph.D. from the City University of New York in 1998 and completed his postdoctoral training at Harvard University in 2001. He then served in the Department of Veterans Affairs of the United States as a principal investigator (2002–2016) in affiliation with the School of Medicine, University of California in Irvine. Currently, he is a professor at Baotou Medical College, Inner Mongolia University of Science and Technology. He has published dozens of research articles on various subjects, including zoology, cardiovascular biology, gastroenterology, and cancer biology. He has been a member of AGA, AHA, ASBMB, and several other professional organizations, and has also served on the editorial board of multiple journals.

Contents

Preface

The esophagus is the long tube running from the back of the mouth to the stomach, and it transports ingested food to the location where real digestion begins. It is a rather simple organ both structurally and functionally, but can be life threatening once it becomes sick, especially when it is malignant. As pointed out in the introductory chapter, "Esophagus and Esophageal Cancer," esophageal cancer kills more than 400,000 people annually and its 5-year survival rate is around 18%. What is even worse, while the incidence of other cancers is declining year after year, esophageal cancer has been moving up steadily for the past several decades, and it casts a really big shadow on the future of human life. Until now there have been no effective drugs to treat esophageal cancer. Most professionals agree that immunotherapy might hold a brighter future in chemotherapy, as demonstrated by the outcomes that have been obtained in several types of cancers. Immunotherapy is a relatively new concept based on immunological principles to battle against cancers, such as activating and orchestrating B-cells and T-cells to attack tumor cells, introducing specific antibodies to induce tumor cell apoptosis, blocking certain signaling pathways to let the tumor cells die of starvation, etc. Chapter 2, "Immunotherapy for Esophageal Cancer," gives a thorough review of this topic, including the history of immunotherapy, drugs that are in use as well as those in trials, and mechanisms of functionality of each drug. It is full of useful information not only for clinicians but also for researchers.

While chemotherapy has been making progress, surgical operation has been a common strategy for esophageal cancer patients. To be exact, during surgery the affected esophagus is cut off partially or entirely. Because of the critical location of the organ, however, the success of surgery often depends greatly on the skills of the operating surgeon. For this reason, robots have been brought into the surgical room in recent years. This has been proven to be at least comparable to a skillful surgeon at this point. Chapter 3, "Robotic Esophageal Surgery for Cancer," tells the story of the actual use of the technology in Germany. Based on experience, this is a promising new way to perform an operation because it can eliminate several human errors. However, a few limitations still exist, such as lack of tactile feedback, longer setup time, and higher overall cost. We believe that these shortcomings can be overcome in the near future, as we continue to improve the system. Even with the help from a robot, post-operative complications are still very common. To reduce such unfortunate chances, proper preparations and care are important not just before surgery, but also during and after surgery. Chapter 4, "Prevention and Management of Complications from Esophagectomy," gives a detailed discussion of this subject, from patient selection to surgeon selection, from assessment of the hospital to a blueprint of the surgical procedure, and more. It also provides advice on how to prevent complications before surgery, as well as how to manage complications when they happen. It discusses six types of complications in particular, including atrial fibrillation, respiratory illness, anastomotic leaks, fistula, delayed gastric emptying, and chyle leaks.

There are two types of esophageal cancer commonly seen. Although esophageal squamous cell carcinoma (ESCC) is the most popular, esophageal adenocarcinoma (EAC) is the fastest growing cancer in the world. While tobacco smoking in conjunction with alcohol consumption might be blamed for causing ESCC, gastroesophageal reflux disease (GERD) has been recognized as the primary reason for the rise of EAC. GERD develops when the lower esophageal sphincter fails to keep the stomach contents from backing into the esophagus. Consequently, the esophageal epithelial lining is frequently exposed to highly acidic stomach fluid that often contains bile salts from the duodenum. When such episodes go on for a long time without proper management, EAC develops. According to recent studies, GERD increases the risk of EAC by 8.6-fold. Currently, GERD is the most common gastrointestinal diagnosis in the United States. Over 60% of Americans experience occasional episodes of acid reflux, and approximately 25% deal with the problem on a weekly basis. Chapter 5, "The Clinical Relevance of Gastroesophageal Reflux Disease and Laryngo-Pharyngeal Reflux in Clinical Practice," is an updated review of GERD clinical practice. It also compares GERD with another abnormality that occurs in close vicinity, lanryngo-pharyngeal reflux (LPR), which is considered as an extra-esophageal manifestation of GERD. Unlike esophageal mucosa, both laryngeal and pharyngeal mucosa do not have sufficient self-protective mechanisms; therefore, the refluxant quickly leads to mucosal lesions. The chapter covers the physiology and pathology of GERD and LPR, as well as their diagnosis and treatment options. It is a good reference for clinical professionals.

Because we are talking about the larynx and pharynx, their malignancies are also commonly treated by surgical operation to remove the troubled organ. Consequently, the patient ends up with loss of vocal ability. To help the patient to maintain minimal voice communication skills, the individual has to be trained to use his/her esophagus as the secondary vocal apparatus, using airflow to cause esophageal mucosa vibration and thereby producing sound. As discussed in Chapter 6, "The Role of Esophagus in Voice Rehabilitation of Laryngectomees," there are two ways to do this: the esophageal speech method and trachea-esophageal speech method. In the esophageal speech method, the respiratory and digestive systems are completely separated. Therefore, the esophagus has to work alone to generate a voice. In the trachea-esophageal speech method, on the other hand, a silicon prosthesis is inserted into the location where the larynx used to be, and connects the respiratory system to the esophagus, so that the patient uses airflow from the lung to vibrate the esophageal mucosa to make a sound. It is a tough job, but there is no other way to deal with the problem at this point.

We have come to a realization that this book might be light by weight, but the subject is quite heavy. Esophageal cancer is the sixth deadliest cancer in the world and could get worse because of the increasing patient population. Through this book, we hope to raise the awareness of health professionals as well as non-professionals, such as politicians and administrators in funding agencies. We need to inject more resources and effort into the battle against this disease.

Jianyuan Chai, Ph.D.
Inner Mongolia Institute of Digestive Diseases
Baotou, China

Chapter 1

Introductory Chapter: Esophagus and Esophageal Cancer

Jianyuan Chai

Additional information is available at the end of the chapter

http://dx.doi.org/10.5772/intechopen.77995

1. Introduction

Our body obtains nutritional supplies from the environment through two primary pipes: bronchus and esophagus, the two simplest organs in the respiratory and digestive systems, respectively. While the bronchus passes oxygen to the lung and expels carbon dioxide out of our biological system, the esophagus transports water and food into the stomach from where a sophisticated process of digestion and nutrient extraction begins.

Although skin cancer might be the most common malignancy in the world, accounting for at least 40% of all cancer cases [1], it is usually excluded from the annual cancer report due to its least perniciousness. The remainders are mostly found in the respiratory and digestive systems, particularly in the digestive system, which hides about twice as much cancer as found in the respiratory system. Five of the top 10 deadliest cancers take place in the digestive organs, including stomach, liver, colon, pancreas, and esophagus. Esophageal cancer is ranked as No. 6 on the list. While the incidence of most cancers is declining year by year, esophageal cancer continues climbing as the fast growing malignancy in the world. Based on a recent prediction, by the year of 2035, the global population of the esophageal cancer patients will be up by 77.4% [2]. In some regions of Asia, Africa, and the South America, the numbers could be doubled in less than 20 years. Logically, esophageal malignancy will very likely become one of the top global concerns in the near future.

The human esophagus is just a short tube of ~25 cm, separating from the rest of the body by two muscular rings at the ends, the upper esophageal sphincter and the lower esophageal sphincter, which control the flow of ingested materials from the mouth to the stomach. Like a corridor that sends visitors from the gate to the main building, the esophagus sends food from the mouth to the stomach. It is a rather simple structure, but, because of its critical location, any abnormalities associated with this organ can be devastating.

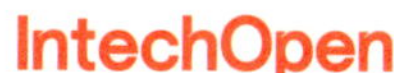

When food is being swallowed, the upper sphincter relaxes, allowing food to enter the pipe. Peristaltic contractions of the esophageal muscle push the food down through the lower sphincter into the stomach. Besides controlling the amount of swallowed food going down into the stomach, the lower esophageal sphincter also works like a dam sitting in between the esophagus and the stomach to prevent the stomach contents to back up into the esophagus. When this muscular structure does not hold well, gastroesophageal reflux disease (GERD) occurs, in which case stomach acid mixed with duodenal content flows back into the esophagus. If this happens frequently enough, it leads to esophagitis, and then to Barret's esophagus, a premalignant metaplasia of the esophageal lining changing from stratified squamous epithelium to simple columnar epithelium. Compared to normal people, individuals with Barret's esophagus can have as high as a 400-fold increased risk to develop esophageal cancer [3].

2. Epidemiology of esophageal cancer

Esophageal cancer is the ninth most common malignancy in the world. Most of the cases are either squamous cell carcinoma (ESCC) or adenocarcinoma (EAC). The former is the predominant one, accounting for ~90% of the cases. ESCC occurs in the squamous cell lining of the middle section of the esophagus and is more often found in Asia and Africa. China alone is responsible for more than 50% of the patient population. EAC, on the other hand, takes place in the cuboidal cells of the esophageal glands near the gastroesophageal junction and has been growing rapidly in western countries in recent years. Both types of esophageal cancer happen more often in males than in females, and the overall ratios of male to female are approximately 2.5 for ESCC and 4.4 for EAC. At the first look, the incidence of esophageal cancer seems to be geographic-related, as ESCC is more seen in Asia and Africa while EAC more common in Europe and North America. However, if we analyze the data further, we notice that the issue is actually more ethnic rather than geographic. Take a look at the cases in the United States, where ESCC incidence is found 4.8 times higher in Asian- and African Americans than in Caucasians, while EAC is just the opposite, 5 times higher in Caucasians than in other Americans [2]. Apparently, these two diseases selectively adhere to certain races of people regardless of where they live. This notion is also supported by the data from China, where ESCC patient population is 77 times greater than that of EAC [4]. Apparently, after a long history of sharing residential resources, each ethnic group has formed its unique life habits. For this reason, they tend to develop common health problems.

As far as we know today, smoking is the No. 1 risk factor for ESCC, particularly when it is in conjunction with drinking. A study found that ESCC incidence increased 12-fold in males and 19-fold in females in the population who use tobacco and alcohol together, compared to those who have one of the hobbies alone [5]. This connection can be easily seen in China, where the tobacco consumption is the highest in the world, higher than all other developing countries combined [6]. The Chinese also consume a lot of alcohol, particularly in northern and central provinces, where the ESCC incidence can reach 0.8% of the local residential population [1]. Here is the east end of the so-called "esophageal cancer belt." This association is also reflected by the data on the American males of Asian and African origins, who tend to smoke and drink abreast, thus making up for 90% of the ESCC patient population in the United States [7].

While the use of tobacco and alcohol together has been the main risk factor for ESCC, obesity and low vegetable consumption increase the chances to develop EAC. In the obese community, the excessive body weight puts constant pressure on the stomach and causes frequent acid reflux. These highly acidic fluids regurgitated from the stomach or even from the duodenum induce inflammation in the esophagus. As the episodes continue, the epithelial lining of the esophagus gradually transforms from stratified squamous epithelium to intestinal columnar phenotype for adaptive protection, as the latter is more endurable to acidic insults. Unfortunately, however, this metaplasia confers a greater danger to become malignant. Studies have shown that people with this kind of esophageal adaptation could have 400 times more likelihood to develop EAC than the general population [8]. Insufficient uptake of fresh fruits and vegetables can also create this type of drama.

Although both ESCC and EAC take place in this short organ, they are very different cancers. From an epidemiological point of view, there is only one common feature between ESCC and EAC, and that is both preferring men over women, while differences are a lot greater.

3. Genetics of esophageal cancer

In addition to the factors associated to life habits, there are also genetic elements contributing to esophageal cancer development. The genomic analysis reveals distinct profiles between ESCC and EAC. ESCC is more similar to squamous cell carcinoma of the head and neck than to EAC, while the latter has more resemblance to gastric adenocarcinoma.

ESCC is believed to develop from basal cell hyperplasia and dysplasia. During this process, the main mutation pattern is C to A substitution, which is commonly found in smokers [9]. The most frequently mutated genes include TP53 (p53, tumor suppression transcription factor), CDKN2A (p16, cyclin-dependent kinase inhibitor), KDM6A (histone demethylase), KMT2D (lysine methyltransferase), and RB1 (retinoblastoma-associated protein). On the other hand, some genes are highly expressed, such as CCND1 (cyclin D1), TP63 (tumor protein), SOX2 (sex-determining region Y), MYC (c-myc), FGFR1 (fibroblast growth factor receptor), TNFAIP3 (tumor necrosis factor-induced protein), and CHN (chimerin) [10]. **Table 1** lists the top five genes frequently mutated and the top five highly expressed.

EAC, on the other hand, is generally believed to originate from Barret's esophagus, an esophageal metaplasia in response to chronic acid reflux. During this process, esophageal epithelium transforms from a multilayer of squamous epithelial cells to a single layer of intestinal columnar epithelial cells, or like the metaphor used by Ahrens et al.: "turning skyscrapers into townhouses" [14]. The natural question is where the columnar cells come from. There are four theories currently to explain the origin of esophageal columnar cells: (1) true trans-differentiation of the esophageal squamous cells, (2) trans-commitment of the esophageal stem cells, (3) colonization and subsequent trans-commitment of bone marrow stem cells, and (4) replacement by gastric columnar epithelial cells.

The first theory is supported by the fact that the esophagus derives from the columnar epithelial cells initially during embryonic development and later is replaced by squamous

Gene	Protein	Function	Up (+)/down (−) in ESCC	References
TP53	p53	Tumor suppression, cellular stress response, cell death	−	[11]
CDKN2A	p16	Stabilizing p53	−	[11, 12]
KDM6A	Lysine demethylase 6A	Chromatin remodeling	−	[9]
KMT2D	Lysine methyltransferase 2D	Chromatin remodeling	−	[9]
RB1	Retinoblastoma transcriptional corepressor 1	Tumor suppression	−	[10]
CCND1	Cyclin D1	Cell cycle progression	+	[9]
TP63	p63	Transcription regulator	+	[9]
SOX2	Sex determining region Y 2	Embryogenesis, stem cell maintenance	+	[9]
MYC	c-myc	Cell cycle progression, cell transformation, apoptosis	+	[9]
EGFR	EGF receptor	Mediating EGF signaling	+	[13]

Table 1. The top five of the most commonly mutated genes (−) and the top five of the most highly expressed genes (+) in ESCC.

epithelium [15]. Therefore, the differentiated esophageal squamous epithelial cells might be able to transform back to columnar cells. Does it sound possible? However, *in vitro* study demonstrated that acid and/or bile treatment upregulated CDX-2 expression in normal esophageal epithelial cells (Het1A), which led to intestinal phenotype [16]. The esophageal epithelium is maintained by a distinct group of p63-expressing stem cells beneath the mucosa under the influence of a specific cue within the organ. When the esophagus is insulted by acidic refluxate repeatedly, the progenitor cells lose p63 expression and are misled to differentiate into columnar instead of squamous epithelial cells. This is where the second theory stands [17]. Does it sound reasonable? More evidence is needed. The third theory seems pretty strong, because it is supported by experimental evidence. In 2008, Sarosi et al. successfully transplanted female rats that had been surgically induced by reflux esophagitis with bone marrow from male rats and later identified Y-chromosome in half of the esophageal epithelial cell population, indicating a colonization of bone marrow stem cells in esophageal epithelium [18]. However, Aikou et al. conducted similar experiment using mice and could not confirm bone marrow-derived metaplastic esophageal epithelial cells [19]. Nevertheless, both the second and third theories recognize the important contribution from stem cells during metaplastic transformation. The only difference is the origin of progenitor cells. If bone marrow stem cells could be misguided to differentiate into columnar phenotype where squamous cells are supposed to be, why could not the local stem cells? The fourth theory has also found experimental evidence in human. In 2014, Lavery et al. showed that labeled gastric cells residing in the middle of esophageal glands had undergone metaplastic transformation, suggesting that esophageal columnar epithelial cells could be from the migration of gastric cardiac columnar epithelial cells [20].

The next question is how esophageal metaplasia turns into EAC. There are two main theories currently. The first theory thinks that EAC develops from Barret's esophagus through a stepwise

Gene	Protein	Function	Up (+)/down (−) in EAC	References
TP53	p53	Tumor suppression, cellular stress response, cell death	−	[21]
CDKN2A	p16	Stabilizing p53	−	[22]
SMAD4	Smad 4	Tumor suppression	−	[23]
SYNE1	Spectrin repeat containing nuclear envelope protein 1	Organelle movement	−	[24]
DOCK2	Dedicator of cytokinesis 2	Cell migration	−	[24]
MYC	c-myc	Cell cycle progression, cell transformation, apoptosis	+	[25]
ERBB2	Her2	Stabilizing EGF binding to its receptor	+	[9]
GATA6	GATA binding protein 6	Cell differentiation in gut	+	[26]
VEGFA	Vascular endothelial growth factor A	Angiogenesis	+	[25]
CCNE1	Cyclin E1	Cell cycle progression	+	[9]

Table 2. The top five of the most commonly mutated genes (−) and the top five of the most highly expressed genes (+) in EAC.

accumulation of gene mutations. EAC is one of cancers with a high rate of gene mutation. In 2013, a study conducted by Dulak et al. performed whole-genome sequence analysis on 149 pairs of EAC versus normal tissue samples and identified a total of 17,383 mutations in 8331 genes in EAC specimens, including 16,516 non-silent mutations and 1954 insertion–deletion-null mutations [24]. Of these genes, 26 were significantly mutated. As seen in ESCC, TP53 and CDKN2A were on top of the list. One of the differences, however, is A to C base transversion that is more common in EAC while C to A is more common in ESCC. The second theory involves a massive chromosomal instability due to the inactivation of p53 and p16. Loss of TP53 has been shown to increase the possibility of malignance by 16-fold [21]. Without functional p53, aneuploidy develops, which increases the pace of genome doubling. CDKN2A is the gene coding for p16, a cyclin-dependent kinase inhibitor that can sequester MDM2 and thereby prevent p53 being degraded. Inactivation of CDKN2A can be interpreted as a reinforcement to the elimination of p53. **Table 2** lists the top five mutated genes and top five overexpressed genes associated with EAC.

4. The guardian of the genome: p53

Based on multiple genetic analyses performed by several independent groups [9, 27–29], TP53 always appeared to be the most frequently mutated gene in both ESCC and EAC. Not just esophageal malignancy, 50–60% of human cancers that have been studied so far contain homozygous mutations in TP53 [30]. That is almost to say, p53 has to be disabled in order to turn a normal cell into a cancerous cell. Why is p53 so important?

TP53 encodes a transcription factor named p53, which has only 393 amino acids. It functions as a tetramer of two dimers, each binding a sequence RRRCWWGYYY (R = A/G, W = A/T, Y = C/T). When a gene contains two such sequences separated by 0–13 base pairs, it becomes a potential target of p53. Up to date, out of 30,000 human genes known so far, 3661 have been found to contain such p53 response elements. In another word, more than 10% of our entire genome is possibly under p53 regulation. Among these target candidates, 346 have been confirmed to be bound and regulated by p53, including 246 upregulated by p53, 91 downregulated by p53, and nine can go either way [31]. That is to say, p53 has the power to shut a gene down or open it up, "all up to its mood."

Normally, after translation, p53 is degraded rapidly through ubiquitination by MDM2, an E3 ubiquitin ligase that happens to be a true target gene of p53. In another word, p53 is a well self-disciplined molecule and can take good care of itself and would not allow itself to accumulate unnecessarily. In response to cellular stresses like DNA damage, oncogene activation, or hypoxia, however, p53 dissociates from MDM2 through various protein modifications such as phosphorylation, acetylation, or methylation, becoming an active transcription factor. Then, p53 rolls out a transcriptional program, namely activating certain genes and/or suppressing some others, to cause cell cycle arrest, senescence, or apoptosis, thereby managing the cellular crisis and bringing the microenvironment back to normal. For this reason, p53 has earned the honor as the "guardian of the genome," and also for this reason, a cell must depower p53 first in order to become malignant.

There are several ways to depower p53 in a cell. Gene mutation is the first one. As mentioned earlier, more than 50% of cancers have TP53 mutations. Interestingly, a majority of these mutations (~ 90%) are missense. In another word, the mutated gene can still be transcribed into a protein product, just different from the wild-type p53. Furthermore, most of these mutations take place at ~190 codons, which encoding the amino acid residues 102–292 within the DNA-binding domain of the transcription factor. Some of the mutant p53 protein products still possess DNA-binding capability to a degree, just weaker, about 0–75% of the wild-type p53 depending on the exact location of the mutation. This is also believed to be the reason for different cancerous phenotypes. Environmental carcinogens tend to cause selective mutations within TP53 and thereby lead to tissue-specific cancers. For instance, tobacco smoke (carcinogen: benzoapyrene diol epoxide) tends to induce mutations at G245 V, G245C, and R249M, which are commonly seen in association with ESCC patients [32]. *In vitro* studies have demonstrated that the expression of mutant p53 in normal cells with TP53 deletion gives them new properties like rapid proliferation, loss of contact inhibition, accelerated migration/invasion, and tumorigenic potential in nude mice, which are the properties that a cancer cell usually possesses, further indicating TP53 mutations in favor of cancer development.

Compared to gene mutation, posttranscriptional regulations also play a significant role in depowering p53. As discussed earlier, p53 protein is constantly degraded by MDM2-mediated ubiquitination. MDM4, a homolog of MDM2, can suppress p53 activation as well, and so do several others, like SIRT1, YY1, MTA2, and HDAC1. Cancer cells learn to cast curses on p53 by overexpressing these proteins in case TP53 mutation did not work. The expression of microRNAs is another example. Several species of microRNAs (i.e., miR-125b, miR-504, and miR-25) have been found to directly bind to p53 mRNA and block it from translation and thereby allow cancer cell to proliferate. By the same principle, microRNAs targeting the suppressors of p53 can indirectly fight for p53 protein stability and activity. For instance, miR-192 increases p53 accumulation by targeting MDM2 mRNA; miR-191 supports p53 stability by blocking MDM4 translation, and miR-34a initiates attacks on YY1 mRNA.

Author details

Jianyuan Chai[1,2]*

*Address all correspondence to: jianyuan.chai@gmail.com

1 Baotou Medical College, Baotou, China

2 School of Medicine, University of California, Irvine, USA

References

[1] Chai J, Jamal MM. Esophageal malignancy: A growing concern. World Journal of Gastroenterology. 2012 Dec 7;**18**(45):6521-6526

[2] Malhotra GK, Yanala U, Ravipati A, Follet M, Vijayakumar M, Are C. Global trends in esophageal cancer. Journal of Surgical Oncology. 2017 Apr;**115**(5):564-579

[3] Chai J. Esophageal Abnormalities. Croatia: Intech Publisher; 2017

[4] Chen W, Sun K, Zheng R, Zeng H, Zhang S, Xia C, Yang Z, Li H, Zou X, He J. Cancer incidence and mortality in China, 2014. Chinese Journal of Cancer Research. 2018;**30**:1-12

[5] Castellsagué X, Muñoz N, De Stefani E, Victora CG, Castelletto R, Rolón PA, Quintana MJ. Independent and joint effects of tobacco smoking and alcohol drinking on the risk of esophageal cancer in men and women. International Journal of Cancer. 1999 Aug 27; **82**(5):657-664

[6] Eriksen MP, Mackay J, Schluger NW, et al. The Tobacco Atlas. Georgia: American Cancer Society Publishing, Atlanta; 2015

[7] Brown LM, Hoover R, Silverman D, Baris D, Hayes R, Swanson GM, Schoenberg J, Greenberg R, Liff J, Schwartz A, Dosemeci M, Pottern L, Fraumeni JF Jr. Excess incidence of squamous cell esophageal cancer among US black men: Role of social class and other risk factors. American Journal of Epidemiology. 2001 Jan 15;**153**(2):114-122

[8] Corley DA. Obesity and the rising incidence of esophageal and gastric adenocarcinoma: What is the link? Gut. 2007;**56**:1493-1494

[9] Cancer Genome Atlas Research Network. Integrated genomic characterization of oesophageal carcinoma. Nature 2017 Jan 12;541(7636):169-175

[10] Lagergren J, Smyth E, Cunningham D, Lagergren P. Esophageal cancer. Lancet. 2017 Nov 25;**390**(10110):2383-2396

[11] Song Y, Li L, Ou Y, Gao Z, Li E, Li X, Zhang W, Wang J, Xu L, Zhou Y, Ma X, Liu L, Zhao Z, Huang X, Fan J, Dong L, Chen G, Ma L, Yang J, Chen L, He M, Li M, Zhuang X, Huang K, Qiu K, Yin G, Guo G, Feng Q, Chen P, Wu Z, Wu J, Ma L, Zhao J, Luo L, Fu M, Xu B, Chen B, Li Y, Tong T, Wang M, Liu Z, Lin D, Zhang X, Yang H, Wang J, Zhan Q. Identification of genomic alterations in oesophageal squamous cell cancer. Nature. 2014 May 1;**509**(7498):91-95

[12] Gao YB, Chen ZL, Li JG, Hu XD, Shi XJ, Sun ZM, Zhang F, Zhao ZR, Li ZT, Liu ZY, Zhao YD, Sun J, Zhou CC, Yao R, Wang SY, Wang P, Sun N, Zhang BH, Dong JS, Yu Y, Luo M, Feng XL, Shi SS, Zhou F, Tan FW, Qiu B, Li N, Shao K, Zhang LJ, Zhang LJ, Xue Q, Gao SG, He J. Genetic landscape of esophageal squamous cell carcinoma. Nature Genetics. 2014 Oct;**46**(10):1097-1102

[13] Smyth EC, Lagergren J, Fitzgerald RC, Lordick F, Shah MA, Lagergren P, Cunningham D. Esophageal cancer. Nature Reviews Disease Primers. 2017 Jul 27;**3**:17048

[14] Ahrens TD, Lutz L, Lassmann S, Werner M. Turning skyscrapers into town houses: Insights into Barrett's esophagus. Pathobiology. 2017;**84**(2):87-98

[15] Mari L, Milano F, Parikh K, Straub D, Everts V, Hoeben KK, Fockens P, Buttar NS, Krishnadath KK. A pSMAD/CDX2 complex is essential for the intestinalization of epithelial metaplasia. Cell Reports. 2014 May 22;**7**(4):1197-1210

[16] Liu T, Zhang X, So CK, Wang S, Wang P, Yan L, Myers R, Chen Z, Patterson AP, Yang CS, Chen X. Regulation of Cdx2 expression by promoter methylation, and effects of Cdx2 transfection on morphology and gene expression of human esophageal epithelial cells. Carcinogenesis. 2007 Feb;**28**(2):488-496

[17] Barbera M, Fitzgerald RC. Cellular origin of Barrett's metaplasia and oesophageal stem cells. Biochemical Society Transactions. 2010 Apr;**38**(2):370-373

[18] Sarosi G, Brown G, Jaiswal K, Feagins LA, Lee E, Crook TW, Souza RF, Zou YS, Shay JW, Spechler SJ. Bone marrow progenitor cells contribute to esophageal regeneration and metaplasia in a rat model of Barrett's esophagus. Diseases of the Esophagus. 2008;**21**(1):43-50

[19] Aikou S, Aida J, Takubo K, Yamagata Y, Seto Y, Kaminishi M, Nomura S. Columnar metaplasia in a surgical mouse model of gastro-esophageal reflux disease is not derived from bone marrow-derived cell. Cancer Science. 2013 Sep;**104**(9):1154-1161

[20] Lavery DL, Nicholson AM, Poulsom R, Jeffery R, Hussain A, Gay LJ, Jankowski JA, Zeki SS, Barr H, Harrison R, Going J, Kadirkamanathan S, Davis P, Underwood T, Novelli MR, Rodriguez-Justo M, Shepherd N, Jansen M, Wright NA, McDonald SA. The stem cell organisation, and the proliferative and gene expression profile of Barrett's epithelium, replicates pyloric-type gastric glands. Gut. 2014 Dec;**63**(12):1854-1863

[21] Reid BJ. p53 and neoplastic progression in Barrett's esophagus. The American Journal of Gastroenterology. 2001 May;**96**(5):1321-1323

[22] Ross-Innes CS, Becq J, Warren A, Cheetham RK, Northen H, O'Donovan M, Malhotra S, di Pietro M, Ivakhno S, He M, Weaver JMJ, Lynch AG, Kingsbury Z, Ross M, Humphray S, Bentley D, Fitzgerald RC. Whole-genome sequencing provides new insights into the clonal architecture of Barrett's esophagus and esophageal adenocarcinoma. Nature Genetics. 2015 Sep;**47**(9):1038-1046

[23] Beroukhim R, Mermel CH, Porter D, Wei G, Raychaudhuri S, Donovan J, Barretina J, Boehm JS, Dobson J, Urashima M, Mc Henry KT, Pinchback RM, Ligon AH, Cho YJ, Haery L, Greulich H, Reich M, Winckler W, Lawrence MS, Weir BA, Tanaka KE, Chiang DY, Bass AJ, Loo A, Hoffman C, Prensner J, Liefeld T, Gao Q, Yecies D, Signoretti S, Maher E, Kaye FJ, Sasaki H, Tepper JE, Fletcher JA, Tabernero J, Baselga J, Tsao MS, Demichelis F, Rubin MA, Janne PA, Daly MJ, Nucera C, Levine RL, Ebert BL, Gabriel S, Rustgi AK, Antonescu CR, Ladanyi M, Letai A, Garraway LA, Loda M, Beer DG, True LD, Okamoto A, Pomeroy SL, Singer S, Golub TR, Lander ES, Getz G, Sellers WR, Meyerson M. The landscape of somatic copy-number alteration across human cancers. Nature. 2010 Feb 18;**463**(7283):899-905

[24] Dulak AM, Stojanov P, Peng S, Lawrence MS, Fox C, Stewart C, Bandla S, Imamura Y, Schumacher SE, Shefler E, McKenna A, Carter SL, Cibulskis K, Sivachenko A, Saksena G, Voet D, Ramos AH, Auclair D, Thompson K, Sougnez C, Onofrio RC, Guiducci C, Beroukhim R, Zhou Z, Lin L, Lin J, Reddy R, Chang A, Landrenau R, Pennathur A, Ogino S, Luketich JD, Golub TR, Gabriel SB, Lander ES, Beer DG, Godfrey TE, Getz G, Bass AJ. Exome and whole-genome sequencing of esophageal adenocarcinoma identifies recurrent driver events and mutational complexity. Nature Genetics. 2013 May;**45**(5):478-486

[25] Dulak AM, Schumacher SE, van Lieshout J, Imamura Y, Fox C, Shim B, Ramos AH, Saksena G, Baca SC, Baselga J, Tabernero J, Barretina J, Enzinger PC, Corso G, Roviello F, Lin L, Bandla S, Luketich JD, Pennathur A, Meyerson M, Ogino S, Shivdasani RA, Beer DG, Godfrey TE, Beroukhim R, Bass AJ. Gastrointestinal adenocarcinomas of the esophagus, stomach, and colon exhibit distinct patterns of genome instability and oncogenesis. Cancer Research 2012 Sep 1;72(17):4383-4393

[26] Pavlov K, Honing J, Meijer C, Boersma-van Ek W, Peters FT, van den Berg A, Karrenbeld A, Plukker JT, Kruyt FA, Kleibeuker JH. GATA6 expression in Barrett's oesophagus and oesophageal adenocarcinoma. Digestive and Liver Disease. 2015 Jan;**47**(1):73-80

[27] Smeenk L, van Heeringen SJ, Koeppel M, Gilbert B, Janssen-Megens E, Stunnenberg HG, Lohrum M. Role of p53 serine 46 in p53 target gene regulation. PLoS One. 2011 Mar 4;**6**(3): e17574

[28] Menendez D, Nguyen TA, Freudenberg JM, Mathew VJ, Anderson CW, Jothi R, Resnick MA. Diverse stresses dramatically alter genome-wide p53 binding and transactivation landscape in human cancer cells. Nucleic Acids Research. 2013 Aug;**41**(15):7286-7301

[29] McDade SS, Patel D, Moran M, Campbell J, Fenwick K, Kozarewa I, Orr NJ, Lord CJ, Ashworth AA, McCance DJ. Genome-wide characterization reveals complex interplay

between TP53 and TP63 in response to genotoxic stress. Nucleic Acids Research. 2014 Jun; **42**(10):6270-6285

[30] Baugh EH, Ke H, Levine AJ, Bonneau RA, Chan CS. Why are there hotspot mutations in the TP53 gene in human cancers? Cell Death and Differentiation. 2017;**2017**:1-7

[31] Fischer M. Census and evaluation of p53 target genes. Oncogene. 2017 Jul 13;**36**(28):3943-3956

[32] Hainaut P, Pfeifer GP. Somatic TP53 mutations in the era of genome sequencing. Cold Spring Harbor Perspectives in Medicine. 2016 Nov 1;**6**(11):1-22

Chapter 2

Immunotherapy for Esophageal Cancer

Tian Wang and Yi Zhang

Additional information is available at the end of the chapter

http://dx.doi.org/10.5772/intechopen.78644

Abstract

As the third most common cancer of the gastrointestinal tract, esophageal cancer has a rather worse prognosis treated with current therapy strategies, and a poor 5-year survival rate lower than 15%. Recent years, emerging immunotherapy has showed a gratifying effect in treating other solid tumors which illuminates its usage for esophageal cancers. Immunotherapy for esophageal cancer basically includes adoptive-cell-therapy-based, antibody-based and vaccine-based therapies, and all of which have shown preliminary favorable results in treating esophageal cancer. However, due to the rather lower mutation rate and a tough microenvironment inside the cancer, promising immunotherapies like immune checkpoint blockade drugs, gene-modified-T cell therapies are hindered by the immunosuppressive factors from microenvironment. Future endeavors will be focusing on targeting immunosuppressive factors, combining immunotherapies with classical treatments to create a satisfying effect.

Keywords: esophageal cancer, tumor microenvironment, immunotherapy, immune checkpoint blockade drugs, CAR-T cell therapy

1. Introduction

Esophageal cancer is one of the leading culprits of mortality worldwide and is responsible for a total number of 746,000 [1] new cases and 439,000 [2] deaths every year. A large number of these cancers are diagnosed at an advanced stage and the metastasis causes bad outcomes. Endoscopic surgery, cytotoxic chemotherapy and radiotherapy remain to be the active and essential clinical treatment but only provide modest benefits, with median overall survival (OS) only in the range of 8–10 months [3]. After nearly 20 years of fast development, immunotherapy turned to be a promising method for treating esophageal cancer. Recent advances have brought some therapeutic regimens to be approved by Food and Drug Administration (FDA) then coming to clinical practice in first- and second-line settings (**Table 1**). The future

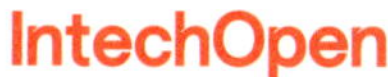

Treatment	Cancer type	Treating method	Phase	Study number
ACT				
	EC	CIK	II	NCT02490735
	Multiple cancer types (including EC)	CTL	I	NCT00004178
	EC	NY-ESO-1-TCR T cells	II	NCT01795976
Tumor vaccine				
Cell vaccine	Multiple cancer types (including EC)	Tumor cell vaccine	I	NCT01258868
	Multiple cancer types (including EC)	H1299 lysate vaccine	I/II	NCT02054104
	Multiple cancer types (including EC)	Allogeneic tumor vaccine	I	NCT01143545
Peptide vaccine	EC	IMF-001	I	NCT01003808
	EC	LY6K, VEGFR1, VEGFR2	I	NCT00561275
	EC	URLC10, TTK, KOC1, VEGFR1, VEGFR2, cisplatin, fluorouracil	I	NCT00632333
	EC	URLC10	I	NCT00753844
	EC, GC	G17DT, cisplatin, fluorouracil	III	NCT00020787
Immune checkpoints therapies	EC + GEJC + GC	Nivolumab/placebo	III	NCT02743494
	EC + GEJC Siewert I	Pembrolizumab vs. investigator's choice	III	NCT02564263
	EC	Pembrolizumab + brachytherapy	I	NCT02642809
	EC	Nivolumab vs. paclitaxel/docetaxel	III	NCT02569242
	EC + GEJC Siewert I	Pembrolizumab	II	NCT02971956
	EC + GC	Pembrolizumab + trastuzumab	II	NCT02318901
	EC	Durvalumab (anti-PD-L1) + chemoradiotherapy	I/II	NCT02735239
	Solid tumors (including ESCC)	LAG525 (anti-LAG3) + PD001 (anti-PD-1)	I/II	NCT02460224
	Solid tumors (including ESCC)	Nivolumab + ipilimumab	I	NCT02834013

ACT: adoptive cell therapy; CIK: cytokine-induced killer cells; CTL: cytotoxic T-cells; VEGFR: vascular endothelial growth factor receptors; PD: programmed cell death receptor; EC: esophageal cancer; ESCC: esophageal squamous cell carcinoma; GEJC: gastroesophageal junction carcinoma.

Table 1. Recent or completed clinical trials of potential therapeutic approaches for immunotherapy of esophageal cancer.

of immunotherapy is promising in treating solid tumors, yet still there is a desperate need for more effective and less toxic treatment options for patients with advanced esophageal cancer.

In recent years, emergence of immunotherapy towards cancer has improved the management of several malignancies dramatically, especially melanoma, renal cell carcinoma, non-small cell lung cancer and so on, shedding light on its usage on esophageal cancer as well. Identification of more suppressive factors in tumor microenvironment and insights into the biology of T cell functioning yielded a large number of diverse and novel anti-tumor regimens. Global efforts continue to explore how and when to integrate these agents in treatment of esophageal cancer. Immune checkpoint inhibition through antibodies that block cytotoxic T-lymphocyte antigen 4 (CTLA-4) and programmed cell death protein 1 (PD-1) has led to meaningful improvements in survival [4]. Vaccine adjuvant administration has also reduced tumor recurrence to some degree. CAR-T (chimeric antigen receptor T-cell) immunotherapy is a typical example of recent advances in synthetic biology, genome engineering, and cell manufacturing that has made it possible to develop highly specific and potent tumor-reactive T cells and offer many opportunities for experimentation and broader clinical translation. Combined regimens of immunotherapy with other classical esophageal treating procedures will illuminate the future of clinical oncotherapy. Recent achievements, which are illustrated below, including finished or ongoing clinical trials and laboratory findings of immunotherapy for esophageal cancer, bringing optimism for meaningful changes in treatment algorithms and for better outcomes in this fatal disease.

2. Immunotherapy regimens for esophageal cancer

2.1. History of immunotherapy

A few decades ago, several rare clinical regression of advanced cancer in response to immune stimulation aroused interests in the area of cancer treatment. A passionate handful of immunologists, oncologists and surgeons carried out forward-looking researches into the relations between tumor progress and body immune system. Their respectable efforts turned the seemingly insignificant clinical phenomenon into reproducible concrete success by revealing the hidden mechanisms of tumor response.

At the earliest period of cancer immunotherapies, the exact mechanism remained unknown and the anti-tumor growth effect was limited yet providing impetus for in-depth study. The first effective immunotherapies aiming at directly modulating cell function using well-characterized recombinant cytokines including interleukin-2 (IL-2) and interferon alpha (IFNα), yet the safety was lowered associated with substantial toxicity. Other cytokines, including IFNγ, IL-4, IL-7, IL-10, IL-12, IL-15, IL-18, IL-25, etc., failed to provide substantive benefit. The following breakthrough was the emerging conception of monoclonal antibodies (mAbs) targeting tumor cell surface receptor proteins (human epidermal growth factor receptor 2 (HER2)/Neu, epidermal growth factor receptor (EGFR), etc.) and were integrated into cancer care. Vaccination therapies using the modified peptide, whole tumor, recombinant proteins, dendritic cells (DCs), and adjuvants were only modestly successful. With researching deeper into the cross-talk happening in the tumor microenvironment between tumor cells and immune cells, the modern era of immunotherapy launched with the extraordinary novel efficacy (and toxicities) of mAbs targeting immune checkpoints in patients with various cancer types in order to decrease the suppressive potential that would prevent immune cells from functioning. Current alternative approach to overcoming the suppressive tumor microenvironment was the administration of genetically modified autologous T cells targeting specific cancer-related antigens [5]. This could be done in the form of T cells in which modified specific T cell receptors (TCR) were inserted for a shared tumor antigen or a tumor-specific neoantigen accompanied by co-transduction of stimulatory cytokines such as IL-12 or could co-administrate with PD-1 pathway blockers to sustain the capability before being expanded in large numbers *in vitro* following lymphodepleting chemotherapy. These approaches have produced dramatic responses in a few patients with a variety of individual tumor types, especially hematological malignancies [6]. Further improvement of adoptive cell transfer therapy came from the modified T cells expressing chimeric antigen receptors (CAR) targeting tumor-specific binding domains. After several generations of amelioration, CAR-T therapy showed extraordinary effect in treating hematological malignancies yet treatment of patients with solid tumors using CAR-T cells had been less fruitful and had troubled clinicians much through the off-tumor/on-target toxicity. Given the virtually limitless possibility of *ex vivo* engineering of T cells, many of these potential hurdles will likely be resolved by the additional modification of T cell products prior to treatment.

Immunotherapy showed great potential in the treatment of esophageal cancer. Modern treatments of patients with esophageal cancer integrated immunotherapy with conventional surgical, chemotherapeutic, and radiation oncologic strategies. In spite of the seemingly gratifying results, the 5-year survival rate of patients with esophageal cancer in the middle and late stages is still lower than 15%, the 5-year survival rate of patients with locally advanced surgery alone is only 20–25% [7]. Postoperative chemotherapy or neoadjuvant chemoradiation only turns the 5-year survival rate up to only 30–35% [8]. One of the causes to blame of the rather poor prognosis of esophageal cancer is the rapid disease progression. More than 50% of patients already have visible metastases at the time of diagnosis [7]. Therefore, further investigation of esophageal cancer microenvironment and its impact on disease progression will lay a solid theoretical foundation for early diagnosis and treatment improvement of esophageal cancer.

In this chapter, we tried to converge concepts relevant to the complicated relationship between the host and the neoplastic tissue.

2.2. Immune microenvironment and molecular correlations in esophageal cancer

As early as 100 years ago, Paget [9] had put forward the hypothesis of "seeds and soil", which laid the foundation for the concept of tumor microenvironment. Numerous data indicate that many immune-related cells, factors and immune-related signaling pathways in the tumor microenvironment play an important role in the occurrence, metastasis, recurrence, angiogenesis, and drug resistance of tumors. The in-depth study of the tumor immune microenvironment is to search for molecular pathogenesis and new therapeutic models of esophageal cancer.

Tumor microenvironment is constituted by various immune cells, endothelial cells, adipocytes, paravascular cells, nerve cells, fibroblasts, and extracellular matrix components around the cancer cells [10]. Some stromal cells in the tumor microenvironment have immunosuppressive potential to inhibit the function of immune effector cells and promote tumor progression. Thus inhibiting cancer cell apoptosis and promoting mechanisms such as proliferation, angiogenesis, drug resistance, and immune escape to promote tumorigenesis [11]. Chemokines CCL17 and CCL22 secreted by tumor cells or tumor-associated macrophages (TAMs) recruit CCR4+ regulatory T cells (Treg), which then inhibit immune effector cells by contacting directly or secretion of cytokines (IL-10 and IL-35). Th17 cells can be transformed into Treg cells stimulated by IL-6 and transforming growth factor-β (TGF-β). Inflammation and tumor-derived factors stimulate the activation of myeloid-derived suppressor cells (MDSCs). Activated MDSCs can directly inhibit the expression of CD8 + T cells. Activation and induction of Treg cells and other mechanisms contribute to immune escape of cancer cells. TAM cells and CAF cells promote the growth, invasion, metastasis, and angiogenesis of tumor cells through the secretion of cytokines, chemokines, and various growth factors. In addition, tumor cells and TAM cells can express programmed cell death ligand (PD)-L1/2 inhibiting T cell activation after binding to PD-1.

MDSCs have been shown to play an important role in promoting tumor immune escape, activating CAF cells and angiogenesis [12]. The presence of proinflammatory cytokines such as IL-1, IL-6 and prostaglandins in esophageal cancer microenvironment can activate MDSC [13]. MDSC inhibits activation of T cells by direct inhibition [14], cytotoxicity of natural killer cells (NK) [15], depletion of arginine and cysteine, induction of Treg cells, etc. to achieve immune escape [16]. Another group of immunosuppressive cells that exert similar functions are Treg cells. Under physiological conditions, Treg cells can regulate the activation and proliferation of T cells, B cells, and cytotoxicity of NK cells. But in tumor microenvironment, Treg cells can promote the occurrence and progression of tumor cells by secreting immunosuppressive related factors, secreting tumor-associated antigens (TAAs), and suppressing the cellular adverse reactions of immune effector cells and the release of granzymes [17]. Studies have shown that tumor cells and TAMs can recruit CCR4+ Treg cells to tumor sites by secreting CCL17 and CCL22 and other chemokines [18]. Treg cells are highly aggregated in tumor cites, promoting tumor invasion and metastasis, and are associated with disease severity, survival after chemotherapy, and prognosis [17]. Additionally, Th17 cells can secrete IL-17 and IL-22 and activate STAT3 related signaling pathways to promote angiogenesis and tumor growth [23]. However, the role of Th17 cells is still controversial. What factors affect the function of Th17 have not yet been well defined [18]. Therefore, we still have to know more about Th17 cells in esophageal cancer to explore potential therapeutic targets.

The tumorigenic mechanisms of TAMs are varied. Phenotype spectrum of macrophage ranges from M1 to M2: M1 macrophages represent the classical activated macrophages, with functions of cytokines secretion, antigen presentation, resistance to infection and anti-tumor ability, etc., while M2 macrophages secrete type II cytokines and induce activation of COX2/prostaglandin E and other mechanisms that cause tumorigenesis [19]. The presence of cancer associated fibroblasts (CAFs) in patients with esophageal cancer is associated with microvessel density, and can also promote tumor progression and metastasis through epithelial mesenchymal transition (EMT). CAFs are also associated with 3-year survival rates and disease recurrence after radiotherapy and chemotherapy [20].

PD-1 is a member of the CD28 superfamily and is an important immunosuppressive molecule that inhibits the activation of T cells after binding to its ligand PD-L1/PD-L2 [4]. Multiple experiments confirmed that PD-L1 and PD-L2 are highly expressed in esophageal cancer [21], in which PD-L1 expression is closely related to tumor invasion depth and poor prognosis, whereas PD-L2 expression is associated with decreased CD8+ T cell infiltration [21]. The increasing PD-L2 expression can promote the secretion of Th2 cytokines such as IL-4/IL-13 [22]. These pieces of evidence suggest that blockers targeting PD-1 are of great significance in the treatment of esophageal cancer [23].

In the early stages of esophageal cancer, TGF-β signaling suppresses tumor growth by down-regulating the expression of Smad4 and c-Myc genes, while promoting growth and EMT in advanced esophageal cancer [24]. This "switching" effect is thought to be caused by the loss of adaptor proteins. For instance, an important adaptor protein, β2-spectrin, plays an important part in cell–cell interactions and maintenance of epithelial cell polarity. In esophageal adenocarcinoma, decreasing β2-spectrin in tumor cells results in increased expression of SOX9 and c-Myc, but it also reduces other TGF-β targets such as E-cadherin and cell cycle-regulated p21 and p27 genes [25]. In summary, these changes make TGF-β promote the progression and metastasis of the tumor by inducing EMT, especially in epithelial tumors like esophageal cancer.

In addition to growth factors, chemokines in the tumor microenvironment also play an important role in the development of tumors. Mainly, there is stromal cell derived factor-1 (CXCL12/SDF-1) secreted by fibroblasts [26], binding to its corresponding receptor CXCR4 or CXCR7 thus inducing tumor growth, promoting angiogenesis, stimulating tumor movement, invasion and metastasis [26]. SDF-1/CXCR4/CXCR7 axis is closely related to tumor invasion, metastasis and survival. However, the use of these separate components as indicators of prognostic analysis has yielded inconsistent results [27]. Nonetheless, CXCL12 has been shown to regulate the migration of CXCR4-positive tumor cells in esophageal adenocarcinoma *in vitro* and *in vivo*. Knockout of CXCR4 expression in KYSE-150 and TE-13 esophageal cancer cells by small interfering RNA can inhibit the proliferation, invasion and metastasis of tumor cells. Local CCL5 and CXCL10 in esophageal squamous cell carcinoma can recruit CD8+ T cells to the tumor site [28].

Further researches showed that remodeling body immune state by various means in esophageal cancer patients will be the main research direction of immunotherapy for esophageal cancer.

2.3. Checkpoint inhibitor regimens

Immune system has sophisticated regulatory mechanisms. Several checkpoints are involved to maintain the balance between effective immune-responses fighting against infection or cancer state yet won't activate excessively to prevent damaging healthy cells. Cytotoxic T lymphocyte antigen-4 (CTLA-4) and PD-1 are among the major inhibitory receptors expressed by Tregs which downregulate immune responses [29]. Inhibitory antibodies modulating these immune checkpoints have been most frequently used in immune-oncology trials in esophageal cancers.

PD-1/PD-L1 blockers have achieved encouraging clinical results in treating melanoma, lung cancer and other cancer types [30, 31]. The potential role of PD-1 blockers in treatment of esophageal cancer can be predicted by genomic map of the tumor immune microenvironment. The expression of PD-L1 on MDSCs isolated from esophageal cancer tissue was higher obviously, and PD-1 expression was detected in approximately 60% of the tumor infiltrating lymphocytes (TILs) from esophageal cancer tissues [32]. Therefore, inhibition of the PD-1/PD-L1 pathway for esophageal cancer treatment cannot be ignored.

Preliminary results of ongoing studies indicated that PD-1 blocker Pembrolizumab had acceptable safety in PD-L1 positive esophageal cancer patients. The objective response rate for mid-term analysis was approximately 30% with a sustained response period of up to 40 weeks [33]. These results laid the foundation for the continued completion of checkpoint inhibitor regimens pivotal study in esophageal cancer patients.

CTLA-4, also known as CD152, belongs to the immunoglobulin superfamily and serves as an immunological checkpoint. When activated CD4+ helper T cells express CTLA-4, this kind of cells sends inhibitory signals to T cells [34]. High CTLA-4 expressing CD4+ Treg cells block T cells by reducing IL-2 secretion and downregulating IL-2 receptor expression then retard T cells in G1 phase of the cell cycle [35]. Ipilimumab and tremelimumab have two fully humanized monoclonal anti-CTLA-4 antibodies that have already received FDA approval for the treatment of melanoma and mesothelioma [36, 37]. A survey of tremelimumab has been completed in phase II clinical trials for treating advanced gastric and esophageal cancer (n = 18). Although only a 5% response rate was observed, four patients were controlled and one patient was observed with partial remission (25.4 Mo) after treatment and continued for several months [38]. The results of ongoing clinical trials are expected to further highlight the clinical value of monoclonal anti-CTLA-4 antibodies in esophageal cancer.

2.4. Vaccine regimens

Tumor vaccine treatment involves the administration of TAAs into patients thus triggering specific anti-tumor immune responses. Rosenberg et al. [39, 40] conducted a comprehensive review of 1306 cancer vaccine usage studies conducted before 2004 and found that the overall target response rate was only 3.3%. The explanation may be that these immune cells have low affinity or are inhibited by endogenous factors like the checkpoints mentioned above.

For the treatment of esophageal cancer, some vaccine-based clinical trial reports have been published. A Phase I clinical trial of 10 patients with refractory stage III or IV esophageal squamous cell carcinoma treated with peptide vaccine found that 9 patients developed antigen-specific T cell immune response. One of the patients with liver metastases showed complete remission for 7 months, another had partial remission within all metastatic lung lesions, and 3 patients had progression-free survival lasting 2.5 months. The peptide vaccine used was derived from three HLA-A24-restricted cancer testis antigens (TTK protein kinase, lymphocyte antigen 6 complex locus K, and insulin-like growth factor-II mRNA binding protein 3) [41]. The multicenter, phase II clinical trial of the vaccine evaluated the OS, PFS, and immune response after vaccinations in patients with HLA-A*2402 positive and negative esophageal squamous cell carcinoma, and immune response was observed in HLA-A*2402 positive patients (n = 35), but there was no statistical difference in OS compared to HLA-A*2402-negative patients (n = 25) (4.6 mo vs. 2.6 mo, P > 0.05), yet there is a significant difference in PFS (P = 0.032) [42]. In a tumor vaccine trial hosted by Saito et al. [43] (n = 20), 4 patients with high levels of MAGE-A4 or MHC class I antigen in autologous tumor cells not only showed MAGE-A4 specific immune responses after vaccination, but compared with patients without using antibodies, their OS was also significantly prolonged. Wada et al. [44] used NY-ESO-1 as a cancer vaccine in 8 patients with esophageal cancer. The results showed that 7 patients had an immune response. Of the 6 patients evaluated for efficacy, 1 patient experienced partial remission, 2 patients continued to maintain progression-free status, and 2 patients had mixed clinical responses. Given the preliminary results of these peptide vaccines in clinical trials, safety inspections and the related researches combined with radiotherapy and chemotherapy are also being carried out gradually in treating multiple cancer types including esophageal cancer.

2.5. Adoptive cell therapy regimens

The concept of ACT (adoptive cell therapy) was first proposed by Dietrich et al. [45]. It refers to the treatment of utilizing autologous or allogeneic immune cells by infusing them back into the patients after being amplified *in vitro* by certain means. Currently effector cells can be divided into two categories: the first type is non-specific immune cells, including autologous lymphokine-activated killer cells (LAK), cytokine-induced killer cells (CIK) and NK cells. Cells are isolated from peripheral blood cells and are stimulated by lymphokines or cytokines; another type of effector cells is antigen-specific T cells, including TILs, cytotoxic T cells (CTL) and genetically engineered T cells including T cell receptor transferred T-cells (TCR-T) and CAR-T [46].

The first ACT trial in human improved the survival of patients with metastatic cancer by reintroduction of CIK and recombinant IL-2 to their body, which has been successfully applied to the treatment of refractory metastatic melanoma, and for other types of cancer such as glioma, renal cell carcinoma, non-small cell lung cancer, etc. The objective response rate varies from 20 to 72% [47], encouraging its further usage in esophageal cancer, too.

So far, ACT treatment of esophageal cancer has been evaluated in several clinical trials. In the first published study by Besser et al. [48] and Toh et al. [49], mononuclear cells were isolated from peripheral blood of esophageal squamous cell carcinoma patients and were given autologous tumor cell stimulation *in vitro*. Latter results showed that half of the patients had an objective response, and 36% of the subjects achieved complete remission or partial remission. CTL and TIL cells are now hot spots for carrying out immunotherapy for solid tumors as the mechanism of killing tumor is rather clear.

TCR-T cells transduce the α and β chains of the antigen-specific high-affinity TCR into T cells and express them on the cell surface, thereby effectively identifying and killing the tumor cells expressing the antigen. Currently, the most common TAAs found in esophageal cancer are cancer testis MAGE-A3/4 and NY-ESO-1. Several studies [50, 51] showed that the expression ratio of MAGE-A3 in esophageal cancer was about 90%, and the expression rate of NYESO-1 in esophageal cancer was up to 40–90%. A preliminary phase 1 clinical trial of genetically engineered T cells was carried out by Kageyama et al. [52], TCR-T cells were readopted to patients with MAGE-A4-positive recurrent esophageal cancer, and administered the MAGE-A4 peptide vaccine subsequently, the level of TCR-T cells in the peripheral blood of 10 subjects was monitored for 5 months, and 5 of them were able to detect specific T cells continuously. Seven subjects appeared tumor progress after 2 months of treatment, but another 3 subjects survived more than 27 months.

CAR-T is another type of genetically engineered T cells. CAR-T was obtained by translocating chimeric antigen receptor such as CARs into T cells. Gross et al. [53] successfully constructed the structure of CARs into T cells for the first time to exert their specific killing function. Up to now, tens of clinical trial data of CAR-T treatment on malignant hematological malignancies have been published. The Novartis' tisagenlecleucel, a synthetic bioimmune product of anti-CD19 CAR-T cells has been approved by FDA on treating relapsed/refractory B-cell acute lymphoblastic leukemia (B-ALL) in 2017 [54]. The early generation of CAR-T therapy for solid tumors did not appear ideal outcomes during clinical use [55]. The reasonable explanation might be lack of unique TAAs in solid tumors, less efficiency and persistency of T cell homing to tumor sites, and the intratumoral immunosuppressive environment strongly inhibited CAR-T cell function. Clinical trials targeting solid tumors using second or third-generation CAR techniques had been limited, but some of the more significant clinical trials are carrying out good results. Patients with metastatic or recurrent HER2-positive medulloblastoma treated with HER2-CAR-T had came out with stable conditions [56]. Feng et al. [57] showed the results of a clinical trial of an EGFR-CAR-T treatment for EGFR-positive relapsed/refractory NSCLC patients revealed partial remission in 2 of the 11 patients involved in the evaluation and 5 patients had a stable condition ranging from 2 to 8 months. There were no obvious adverse reactions in the entire clinical trial. In the treatment of esophageal cancer, no CAR-T therapy-related studies have been conducted yet. However, anti-tumor targets are now erupting in esophageal cancer. Points such as HER2 can also provide references for future steps in the development of research.

3. Combined treatment

Currently, comprehensive therapy shed light on tumor treatment to a large degree. Clinical practice has proven that it is difficult to achieve the best results with any single treatment method. Therefore, the principle of treatment for most tumors depends on comprehensive treatment. Recent research results showed that the combined usage of immunotherapy and chemotherapy in a variety of cancer treatment achieved better results than a single therapy, it can not only reverse the immunosuppression effects caused by the late stage of the tumor, increase the cross-presentation of tumor antigens, promote the proliferation of killer T cells and make it more easy to kill tumor cells, but can also reduce the incidence of adverse reactions from chemotherapy and reduce drug resistance of tumor cells to some extent. Combination of chemotherapy and immunotherapy has been a common available method in some cancer types. Neoadjuvant chemotherapy regimens together with HER2-targeted therapy achieved pathologic complete response in relapse-free survival among patients with breast cancer [58].

New treatment targeting specific mutant genes illustrated clinical success in a phase II study of metastatic melanoma combined with interleukin-2 aldesleukin and BRAF inhibitor vemurafenib [59]. The effectiveness of combined therapy can even cover the metastatic areas, in melanoma brain metastases, complete intracranial response was observed after using dual checkpoint-inhibition of talimogene laherparepvec (T-Vec), pembrolizumab and whole brain radiotherapy. Additionally, immunotherapy also showed potential augmented effect plus cryotherapy [60], focused ultrasound therapy [61] and photothermal therapy [62], etc. Tumor vaccine also took another leap when combined with other immunotherapies, clinical results showed that nivolumab in combination with talimogene laherparepvec (T-Vec) in resected melanoma carried out better outcomes [63]. The clinical value of immunotherapy and radiotherapy showed even more outstanding clinical effects, anti-tumor immune response was enhanced by anti-PD-1 immunotherapy in recurrent nasopharyngeal carcinoma, showing a bright prospect of further combination [64]. In treating esophageal cancer, there are also many creative comprehensive treatment methods that are constantly developing. In patients with drug-resistant esophageal cancer, a phase Ib/II study of low-dose decitabine-primed chemoimmunotherapy showed undeniable safety and efficacy [65]. A combination therapy of multi-peptide vaccine with chemoradiation therapy performed satisfying safety thus can be an effective treatment for patients with unresectable ESCC [66]. Novel multitarget tyrosine kinase inhibitor anlotinib in a third-line treatment of refractory advanced non-small-cell lung cancer (RA-NSCLC) provided significant PFS benefits compared with placebo, and accompanied with acceptable toxicity [67]. Though has a guaranteed future, there need to be more rational and effective trials of combinations to be excavated in the field of treating esophageal cancer together with other solid tumors.

4. Conclusions and future directions

The success of immunotherapy in some tumors came from years of research deep into the immune system and tumor itself and brought hope of healing cancer. It is worth mentioning that several immune checkpoint blockers have been or are being approved by the FDA, and it is expected that the next step will be to accelerate the pace of application of single drug or other treatment modes in combination within clinical usage. However, opportunities and challenges coexist, and there are still some key questions that have not been answered in immunotherapy. First of all, many targeted cancer drugs that treat cancer need to be explored to determine the biological dose that achieves the greatest clinical benefit with minimal toxicity. Second, given that most of the current immunotherapy is mainly to activate anti-tumor effects by activating the immune system, this kind of treatment requires patient to have some degree of immunity before receiving the initial immunotherapy. Therefore, it is imperative to fully evaluate patient's immune status and find biomarkers that predict the effectiveness of immunotherapy. In addition, there is abundant evidence that exposure to radiation and chemotherapy drugs may affect the rate of DNA mutations in tumor cells, prompting the formation of some new antigens. As the current immunotherapy is always combined with radiotherapy and chemotherapy, determining the proper dose for each regimen is the prerequisite for maximum benefit of combined therapy.

Immunotherapy has a broad application prospect in the treatment of malignant tumors. The high frequency of esophageal cancer mutations and the effective results of immunotherapy highlighted in other gastrointestinal cancers provide strong evidence for the study of esophageal cancer immunotherapy. Treatment strategies combined with existing or new treatment modes will be the direction of future esophageal cancer treatment.

Author details

Tian Wang and Yi Zhang*

*Address all correspondence to: yizhang@zzu.edu.cn

Biotherapy Center, The First Affiliated Hospital of Zhengzhou University, Zhengzhou, Henan, China

References

[1] GBD 2015 Disease and Injury Incidence and Prevalence, Collaborators. Lancet. 2016; **388**(10053):1545-1602. DOI: 10.1016/S0140-6736(16)31678-6. PMC: 5055577 PMID: 277-33282

[2] GBD 2015 Mortality and Causes of Death, Collaborators. Lancet. 2016;**388**(10053): 1459-1544. DOI: 10.1016/s0140-6736(16)31012-1. PMC: 5388903 PMID: 27733281

[3] Chang S, Kohrt H, Maecker HT. Monitoring the immune competence of cancer patients to predict outcome. Cancer Immunology, Immunotherapy. 2014;**63**:713-719. DOI: 10. 1007/s00262-014-1521-3. PMID: 24487923

[4] Smyth E, Thuss-Patience PC. Immune checkpoint inhibition in gastro-oesophageal cancer. Oncology Research and Treatment. 2018;**41**(5):272-280. DOI: 10.1159/000489099. PMID: 29705787

[5] Li F, Zhang T, Cao L, Zhang Y. Chimeric antigen receptor T cell based immunotherapy for cancer. Current Stem Cell Research & Therapy. 2018 Apr 19. DOI: 10.2174/1574888X 13666180420110239. PMID: 29676233

[6] Kueberuwa G, Kalaitsidou M, Cheadle E, Hawkins RE, Gilham DE. CD19 CAR T cells expressing IL-12 eradicate lymphoma in fully lymphoreplete mice through induction of host immunity. Molecular Therapy—Oncolytics. 2017 Dec 19;**8**:41-51. DOI: 10.1016/j. omto.2017.12.003 eCollection 2018 Mar 30. PMID: 29367945

[7] Enzinger PC, Mayer RJ. Esophageal cancer. The New England Journal of Medicine. 2003;**349**:2241-2252. DOI: 10.1056/NEJMra035010 PMID: 14657432

[8] Rubenstein JH, Shaheen NJ. Epidemiology, diagnosis, and management of esophageal adenocarcinoma. Gastroenterology. 2015;**149**:302-17.e1. DOI: 10.1053/j.gastro.2015.04.053 PMID: 25957861

[9] Paget S. The distribution of secondary growths in cancer of the breast. 1889. Cancer Metastasis Reviews. 1989;**8**:98-101 PMID: 2673568

[10] Karakasheva TA, Dominguez GA, Hashimoto A, Lin EW, Chiu C, Sasser K, Lee JW, Beatty GL, Gabrilovich DI, Rustgi AK. CD38+ M-MDSC expansion characterizes a subset of advanced colorectal cancer patients. JCI Insight. 2018 Mar 22;**3**(6):pii-97022. DOI: 10.1172/jci.insight.97022 PMID: 29563330

[11] Whiteside TL. The tumor microenvironment and its role in promoting tumor growth. Oncogene. 2008;**27**:5904-5912. DOI: 10.1038/onc.2008.271 PMID: 18836471

[12] Zhu Y, Zhang L, Zha H, Yang F, Hu C, Chen L, Guo B, Zhu B. Stroma-derived fibrinogen-like protein 2 activates cancer-associated fibroblasts to promote tumor growth in lung cancer. International Journal of Biological Sciences. 2017 Jun 1;**13**(6):804-814. DOI: 10.7150/ijbs.19398 eCollection 2017. PMID: 28656005

[13] Okano S, Abu-Elmagd K, Kish DD, Keslar K, Baldwin WM 3rd, Fairchild RL, Fujiki M, Khanna A, Osman M, Costa G, Fung J, Miller C, Kayashima H, Hashimoto K. Myeloid-derived suppressor cells increase and inhibit donor-reactive T cell responses to graft intestinal epithelium in intestinal transplant patients. American Journal of Transplantation. 2018 Mar 6. DOI: 10.1111/ajt.14718. PMID: 29509288

[14] Parker KH, Beury DW, Ostrand-Rosenberg S. Myeloid-derived suppressor cells: Critical cells driving immune suppression in the tumor microenvironment. Advances in Cancer Research. 2015;**128**:95-139. DOI: 10.1016/bs.acr.2015.04.002

[15] Spallanzani RG1, Dalotto-Moreno T, Raffo Iraolagoitia XL, Ziblat A, Domaica CI, Avila DE, Rossi LE, Fuertes MB, Battistone MA, Rabinovich GA, Salatino M, Zwirner NW. Expansion of CD11b(+)Ly6G (+)Ly6C (int) cells driven by medroxyprogesterone acetate in mice bearing breast tumors restrains NK cell effector functions. Cancer Immunology, Immunotherapy. 2013 Dec;**62**(12):1781-1795. DOI: 10.1007/s00262-013-1483-x. PMID: 24114144

[16] Fleming V, Hu X, Weber R, Nagibin V, Groth C, Altevogt P, Utikal J, Umansky V. Targeting myeloid-derived suppressor cells to bypass tumor-induced Immunosuppression. Frontiers in Immunology. 2018 Mar 2;**9**:398. DOI: 10.3389/fimmu.2018.00398 eCollection 2018. PMID: 29552012

[17] Ahrends T, Borst J. The opposing roles of CD4+ T cells in anti-tumor immunity. Immunology. 2018 Apr 27. DOI: 10.1111/imm.12941. PMID: 29700809

[18] Yang G, Li H, Yao Y, Xu F, Bao Z, Zhou J. Treg/Th17 imbalance in malignant pleural effusion partially predicts poor prognosis. Oncology Reports. 2015 Jan;**33**(1):478-484. DOI: 10.3892/or.2014.3576

[19] Wang Y, Xu G, Wang J, Li XH, Sun P, Zhang W, Li JX, Wu CY. Relationship of Th17/Treg cells and radiation pneumonia in locally advanced esophageal carcinoma. Anticancer Research. 2017 Aug;**37**(8):4643-4647

[20] Qiao Y, Zhang C, Li A, Wang D, Luo Z, Ping Y, Zhou B, Liu S, Li H, Yue D, Zhang Z, Chen X, Shen Z, Lian J, Li Y, Wang S, Li F, Huang L, Wang L, Zhang B, Yu J, Qin Z, Zhang Y. IL6 derived from cancer-associated fibroblasts promotes chemoresistance via CXCR7 in esophageal squamous cell carcinoma. Oncogene. 2018 Feb 15;**37**(7):873-883. DOI: 10.1038/onc.2017.387

[21] Guo W, Wang P, Li N, Shao F, Zhang H, Yang Z, Li R, Gao Y, He J. Prognostic value of PD-L1 in esophageal squamous cell carcinoma: A meta-analysis. Oncotarget. 2017 Dec 27;**9**(17):13920-13933. DOI: 10.18632/oncotarget.23810. PMID: 29568405

[22] Freeman GJ, Long AJ, Iwai Y, Bourque K, Chernova T, Nishimura H, Fitz LJ, Malenkovich N, Okazaki T, Byrne MC, Horton HF, Fouser L, Carter L, Ling V, Bowman MR, Carreno BM, Collins M, Wood CR, Honjo T. Engagement of the PD-1 immunoinhibitory receptor by a novel B7 family member leads to negative regulation of lymphocyte activation. The Journal of Experimental Medicine. 2000;**192**:1027-1034. DOI: 10.1084/jem.192.7.1027. PMID: 11015443

[23] Walsh EM, Kelly RJ. Single agent anti PD-1 inhibitors in esophageal cancer—A first step in a new therapeutic direction. Journal of Thoracic Disease. 2018 Mar;**10**(3):1308-1313. DOI: 10.21037/jtd.2018.03.43

[24] Caja L, Dituri F, Mancarella S, Caballero-Diaz D, Moustakas A, Giannelli G, Fabregat I. TGF-β and the tissue microenvironment: Relevance in fibrosis and cancer. International Journal of Molecular Sciences. 2018 Apr 26;**19**(5). DOI: 10.3390/ijms19051294

[25] Song S, Maru DM, Ajani JA, Chan CH, Honjo S, Lin HK, Correa A, Hofstetter WL, Davila M, Stroehlein J, Mishra L. Loss of TGF-β adaptor 2SP activates notch signaling and SOX9 expression in esophageal adenocarcinoma. Cancer Research. 2013;**73**:2159-2169. DOI: 10.1158/0008-5472.CAN-12-1962

[26] Givel AM, Kieffer Y, Scholer-Dahirel A, Sirven P, Cardon M, Pelon F, Magagna I, Gentric G, Costa A, Bonneau C, Mieulet V, Vincent-Salomon A, Mechta-Grigoriou F. miR200-regulated CXCL12β promotes fibroblast heterogeneity and immunosuppression in ovarian cancers. Nature Communications. 2018 Mar 13;**9**(1):1056. DOI: 10.1038/s41467-018-03348-z

[27] Nazari A, Khorramdelazad H, Hassanshahi G. Biological/pathological functions of the CXCL12/CXCR4/CXCR7 axes in the pathogenesis of bladder cancer. International Journal of Clinical Oncology. 2017 Dec;**22**(6):991-1000. DOI: 10.1007/s10147-017-1187-x. PMID: 29022185

[28] Liu J, Li F, Ping Y, Wang L, Chen X, Wang D, Cao L, Zhao S, Li B, Kalinski P, Thorne SH, Zhang B, Zhang Y. Local production of the chemokines CCL5 and CXCL10 attracts CD8+ T lymphocytes into esophageal squamous cell carcinoma. Oncotarget. 2015;**6**: 24978-24989. DOI: 10.18632/oncotarget.4617

[29] Liu Z, McMichael EL, Shayan G, Li J, Chen K, Srivastava RM, Kane LP, Lu B, Ferris RL. Novel effector phenotype of Tim-3+ regulatory T cells leads to enhanced suppressive

function in head and neck cancer patients. Clinical Cancer Research. 2018 Apr 30. DOI: 10.1158/1078-0432.CCR-17-1350. PMID: 29712685

[30] Borghaei H, Paz-Ares L, Horn L, Spigel DR, Steins M, Ready NE, Chow LQ, Vokes EE, Felip E, Holgado E, Barlesi F, Kohlhäufl M, Arrieta O, Burgio MA, Fayette J, Lena H, Poddubskaya E, Gerber DE, Gettinger SN, Rudin CM, Rizvi N, Crinò L, Blumenschein GR, Antonia SJ, Dorange C, Harbison CT, Graf Finckenstein F, Brahmer JR. Nivolumab versus docetaxel in advanced nonsquamous non-small-cell lung cancer. The New England Journal of Medicine. 2015;**373**:1627-1639. DOI: 10.1056/NEJMoa1507643. PMID: 26412456

[31] Long GV, Atkinson V, Lo S, Sandhu S, Guminski AD, Brown MP, Wilmott JS, Edwards J, Gonzalez M, Scolyer RA, Menzies AM, McArthur GA. Combination nivolumab and ipilimumab or nivolumab alone in melanoma brain metastases: A multicentre randomised phase 2 study. The Lancet Oncology. 2018 Mar 27. DOI: 10.1016/S1470-2045(18)30139-6. PMID: 29602646

[32] Huang H, Zhang G, Li G, Ma H, Zhang X. Circulating CD14(+)HLA-DR(−/low) myeloid-derived suppressor cell is an indicator of poor prognosis in patients with ESCC. Tumour Biology. 2015;**36**:7987-7996. DOI: 10.1007/s13277-015-3426-y. PMID: 25967454

[33] Doi T, Piha-Paul SA, Jalal SI, Saraf S, Lunceford J, Koshiji M, Bennouna J. Safety and antitumor activity of the anti-programmed death-1 antibody pembrolizumab in patients with advanced esophageal carcinoma. Journal of Clinical Oncology. 2018 Jan 1;**36**(1): 61-67. DOI: 10.1200/JCO.2017.74.9846

[34] Santoni G, Amantini C, Morelli MB, Tomassoni D, Santoni M, Marinelli O, Nabissi M, Cardinali C, Paolucci V, Torniai M, Rinaldi S, Morgese F, Bernardini G, Berardi R. High CTLA-4 expression correlates with poor prognosis in thymoma patients. Oncotarget. 2018 Mar 30;**9**(24):16665-16677. DOI: 10.18632/oncotarget.24645. eCollection 2018 Mar 30

[35] Liu D, Badell IR, Ford ML. Selective CD28 blockade attenuates CTLA-4-dependent CD8+ memory T cell effector function and prolongs graft survival. JCI Insight. 2018 Jan 11;**3**(1). DOI: 10.1172/jci.insight.96378 PMID: 29321374

[36] Diao K, Bian SX, Routman DM, Yu C, Ye JC, Wagle NA, Wong MK, Zada G, Chang EL. Stereotactic radiosurgery and ipilimumab for patients with melanoma brain metastases: Clinical outcomes and toxicity. Journal of Neuro-Oncology. 2018 Apr 25. DOI: 10.1007/s11060-018-2880-y. PMID: 29696531

[37] Maio M, Scherpereel A, Calabrò L, Aerts J, Cedres Perez S, Bearz A, Nackaerts K, Fennell DA, Kowalski D, Tsao AS, Taylor P, Grosso F, Antonia SJ, Nowak AK, Taboada M, Puglisi M, Stockman PK, Kindler HL. Tremelimumab as second-line or third-line treatment in relapsed malignant mesothelioma (DETERMINE): A multicentre, international, randomised, double-blind, placebo-controlled phase 2b trial. The Lancet Oncology. 2017 Sep;**18**(9):1261-1273. DOI: 10.1016/S1470-2045(17)30446-1 Epub 2017 Jul 17. PMID: 28729154

[38] Ralph C, Elkord E, Burt DJ, O'Dwyer JF, Austin EB, Stern PL, Hawkins RE, Thistlethwaite FC. Modulation of lymphocyte regulation for cancer therapy: A phase II trial of tremelimumab in advanced gastric and esophageal adenocarcinoma. Clinical Cancer Research. 2010;**16**:1662-1672. DOI: 10.1158/1078-0432.CCR-09-2870. PMID: 20179239

[39] Rosenberg SA, Yang JC, Restifo NP. Cancer immunotherapy: Moving beyond current vaccines. Nature Medicine. 2004;**10**:909-915. DOI: 10.1038/nm1100. PMID: 15340416

[40] Rosenberg SA, Sherry RM, Morton KE, Scharfman WJ, Yang JC, Topalian SL, Royal RE, Kammula U, Restifo NP, Hughes MS, Schwartzentruber D, Berman DM, Schwarz SL, Ngo LT, Mavroukakis SA, White DE, Steinberg SM. Tumor progression can occur despite the induction of very high levels of self/tumor antigen-specific CD8+ T cells in patients with melanoma. Journal of Immunology. 2005;**175**:6169-6176. DOI: 10.4049/jimmunol.175.9.6169. PMID: 16237114

[41] Kono K, Mizukami Y, Daigo Y, Takano A, Masuda K, Yoshida K, Tsunoda T, Kawaguchi Y, Nakamura Y, Fujii H. Vaccination with multiple peptides derived from novel cancer-testis antigens can induce specific T-cell responses and clinical responses in advanced esophageal cancer. Cancer Science. 2009;**100**:1502-1509. DOI: 10.1111/j.1349-7006.2009.01200.x. PMID: 19459850

[42] Kono K, Iinuma H, Akutsu Y, Tanaka H, Hayashi N, Uchikado Y, Noguchi T, Fujii H, Okinaka K, Fukushima R, Matsubara H, Ohira M, Baba H, Natsugoe S, Kitano S, Takeda K, Yoshida K, Tsunoda T, Nakamura Y. Multicenter, phase II clinical trial of cancer vaccination for advanced esophageal cancer with three peptides derived from novel cancer-testis antigens. Journal of Translational Medicine. 2012;**10**:141. DOI: 10.1186/1479-5876-10-141. PMID: 22776426

[43] Saito T, Wada H, Yamasaki M, Miyata H, Nishikawa H, Sato E, Kageyama S, Shiku H, Mori M, Doki Y. High expression of MAGE-A4 and MHC class I antigens in tumor cells and inductionof MAGE-A4 immune responses are prognostic markers of CHP-MAGE-A4 cancer vaccine. Vaccine. 2014;**32**:5901-5907. DOI: 10.1016/j.vaccine.2014.09.002. PMID: 25218300

[44] Wada H, Sato E, Uenaka A, Isobe M, Kawabata R, Nakamura Y, Iwae S, Yonezawa K, Yamasaki M, Miyata H, Doki Y, Shiku H, Jungbluth AA, Ritter G, Murphy R, Hoffman EW, Old LJ, Monden M, Nakayama E. Analysis of peripheral and local anti-tumor immune response in esophageal cancer patients after NY-ESO-1 protein vaccination. International Journal of Cancer. 2008;**123**:2362-2369. DOI: 10.1002/ijc.23810. PMID: 18729190

[45] Dietrich A, Mitchison NA, Rajnavölgyi E, Schneider SC. Primed lymphocytes are boosted by type II collagen of their hosts after adoptive transfer. Journal of Autoimmunity. 1994;**7**:601-609. DOI: 10.1006/jaut.1994.1044. PMID: 7840853

[46] Alsina M, Moehler M, Lorenzen S. Immunotherapy of esophageal cancer: Current status, many trials and innovative strategies. Oncology Research and Treatment. 2018;**41**(5): 266-271. DOI: 10.1159/000488120. Epub 2018 Apr 20

[47] Rosenberg SA, Lotze MT, Muul LM, Leitman S, Chang AE, Ettinghausen SE, Matory YL, Skibber JM, Shiloni E, Vetto JT. Observations on the Systemic Administration of Autologous Lymphokine-Activated Killer Cells and Recombinant Interleukin-2 to Patients with Metastatic Cancer

[48] Besser MJ, Shapira-Frommer R, Schachter J. Tumor-infiltrating lymphocytes: Clinical experience. Cancer Journal. 2015;**21**:465-469 PMID: 26588677. DOI: 10.1097/PPO.0000-000000000154

[49] Toh U, Yamana H, Sueyoshi S, Tanaka T, Niiya F, Katagiri K, Fujita H, Shirozou K, Itoh K. Locoregional cellular immunotherapy for patients with advanced esophageal cancer. Clinical Cancer Research. 2000;**6**:4663-4673. PMID: 11156218

[50] Chen X, Wang L, Yue D, Liu J, Huang L, Yang L, Cao L, Qin G, Li A, Wang D, Wang M, Qi Y, Zhang B, van der Bruggen P, Zhang Y. Correlation between the high expression levels of cancer-germline genes with clinical characteristics in esophageal squamous cell carcinoma. Histology and Histopathology. 2017 Aug;**32**(8):793-803. DOI: 10.14670/HH-11-847. Epub 2016 Nov 21

[51] Bujas T, Marusic Z, Peric Balja M, Mijic A, Kruslin B, Tomas D. MAGE-A3/4 and NY-ESO-1 antigens expression in metastatic esophageal squamous cell carcinoma. European Journal of Histochemistry. 2011;**55**:e7. DOI: 10.4081/ejh. 2011.e7. PMID: 21556122

[52] Kageyama S, Wada H, Muro K, Niwa Y, Ueda S, Miyata H, Takiguchi S, Sugino SH, Miyahara Y, Ikeda H, Imai N, Sato E, Yamada T, Osako M, Ohnishi M, Harada N, Hishida T, Doki Y, Shiku H. Dose-dependent effects of NY-ESO-1 protein vaccine complexed with cholesteryl pullulan (CHP-NY-ESO-1) on immune responses and survival benefits of esophageal cancer patients. Journal of Translational Medicine. 2013;**11**:246. DOI: 10.1186/1479-5876-11-246. PMID: 24093426

[53] Gross G, Waks T, Eshhar Z. Expression of immunoglobulin-T-cell receptor chimeric molecules as functional receptors with antibodytype specificity. Proceedings of the National Academy of Sciences of the United States of America. 1989;**86**:10024-10028. DOI: 10.1073/pnas.86.24.10024. PMID: 2513569

[54] Liu Y, Chen X, Han W, Zhang Y. Tisagenlecleucel, an approved anti-CD19 chimeric antigen receptor T-cell therapy for the treatment of leukemia. Drugs Today (Barc). 2017 Nov;**53**(11):597-608. DOI: 10.1358/dot.2017.53.11.2725754. PMID: 29451276

[55] Kershaw MH, Westwood JA, Parker LL, Wang G, Eshhar Z, Mavroukakis SA, White DE, Wunderlich JR, Canevari S, Rogers-Freezer L, Chen CC, Yang JC, Rosenberg SA, Hwu P. A phase I study on adoptive immunotherapy using gene-modified T cells for ovarian cancer. Clinical Cancer Research. 2006;**12**:6106-6115. DOI: 10.1158/1078-0432.CCR-06-1183. PMID: 17062687

[56] Nellan A, Rota C, Majzner R, Lester-McCully CM, Griesinger AM, Mulcahy Levy JM, Foreman NK, Warren KE, Lee DW. Durable regression of Medulloblastoma after regional

and intravenous delivery of anti-HER2 chimeric antigen receptor T cells. Journal for Immunotherapy of Cancer. 2018 Apr 30;**6**(1):30. DOI: 10.1186/s40425-018-0340-z

[57] Feng K, Guo Y, Dai H, Wang Y, Li X, Jia H, Han W. Chimeric antigen receptor-modified T cells for the immunotherapy of patients with EGFR expressing advanced relapsed/refractory nonsmall cell lung cancer. Science China. Life Sciences. 2016;**59**:468-479. DOI: 10.1007/s11427-016-5023-8. PMID: 26968708

[58] Weiss A, Bashour SI, Hess K, Thompson AM, Ibrahim NK. Effect of neoadjuvant chemotherapy regimen on relapse-free survival among patients with breast cancer achieving a pathologic complete response: An early step in the de-escalation of neoadjuvant chemotherapy. Breast Cancer Research. 2018;**20**:27. DOI: 10.1186/s13058-018-0945-7

[59] Mooradian MJ, Reuben A, Prieto PA, Hazar-Rethinam M, Frederick DT, Nadres B, Piris A, Juneja V, Cooper ZA, Sharpe AH, Corcoran RB, Flaherty KT, Lawrence DP, Wargo JA, Sullivan RJ. A phase II study of combined therapy with a BRAF inhibitor (vemurafenib) and interleukin-2 (aldesleukin) in patients with metastatic melanoma. Oncoimmunology. 2018 Feb 1;**7**(5):e1423172. DOI: 10.1080/2162402X.2017.1423172. eCollection 2018

[60] Abdo J, Cornell DL, Mittal SK, Agrawal DK. Immunotherapy plus cryotherapy: Potential augmented abscopal effect for advanced cancers. Frontiers in Oncology. 2018 Mar 28;**8**:85. DOI: 10.3389/fonc.2018.00085. eCollection 2018

[61] Mauri G, Nicosia L, Xu Z, Di Pietro S, Monfardini L, Bonomo G, Varano GM, Prada F, Della Vigna P, Orsi F. Focused ultrasound: Tumour ablation and its potential to enhance immunological therapy to cancer. The British Journal of Radiology. 2018 Feb;**91**(1083):20170641. DOI: 10.1259/bjr.20170641

[62] Mi FL, Burnouf T, Lu SY, Lu YJ, Lu KY, Ho YC, Kuo CY, Chuang EY. Self-targeting, immune transparent plasma protein coated nanocomplex for noninvasive photothermal anticancer therapy. Advanced Healthcare Materials. 2017 Jul;**6**(14). DOI: 10.1002/adhm.201700181

[63] Blake Z, Marks DK, Gartrell RD, Hart T, Horton P, Cheng SK, Taback B, Horst BA, Saenger YM. Complete intracranial response to talimogene laherparepvec (T-Vec), pembrolizumab and whole brain radiotherapy in a patient with melanoma brain metastases refractory to dual checkpoint-inhibition. Journal for Immunotherapy of Cancer. 2018 Apr 6;**6**(1):25. DOI: 10.1186/s40425-018-0338-6

[64] Finazzi T, Rordorf T, Ikenberg K, Huber GF, Guckenberger M, Schueler G, HI. Radiotherapy-induced anti-tumor immune response and immune-related adverse events in a case of recurrent nasopharyngeal carcinoma undergoing anti-PD-1 immunotherapy. BMC Cancer. 2018 Apr 6;**18**(1):395. DOI: 10.1186/s12885-018-4295-8

[65] Chen M, Nie J, Liu Y, Li X, Zhang Y, Brock MV, Feng K, Wu Z, Li X, Shi L, Li S, Guo M, Mei Q, Han W. Phase Ib/II study of safety and efficacy of low-dose decitabine-primed chemoimmunotherapy in patients with drug-resistant relapsed/refractory alimentary tract cancer. International Journal of Cancer. 2018 Apr 16. DOI: 10.1002/ijc.31531

[66] Iinuma H, Fukushima R, Inaba T, Tamura J, Inoue T, Ogawa E, Horikawa M, Ikeda Y, Matsutani N, Takeda K, Yoshida K, Tsunoda T, Ikeda T, Nakamura Y, Okinaga K. Phase I clinical study of multiple epitope peptide vaccine combined with chemoradiation therapy in esophageal cancer patients. Journal of Translational Medicine. 2014 Apr 3;**12**:84. DOI: 10.1186/1479-5876-12-84

[67] Han B, Li K, Zhao Y, Li B, Cheng Y, Zhou J, Lu Y, Shi Y, Wang Z, Jiang L, Luo Y, Zhang Y, Huang C, Li Q, Wu G. Anlotinib as a third-line therapy in patients with refractory advanced non-small-cell lung cancer: A multicentre, randomised phase II trial (ALTER0302). British Journal of Cancer. 2018 Mar 6;**118**(5):654-661. DOI: 10.1038/bjc.2017.478

Chapter 3

Prevention and Management of Complications from Esophagectomy

Jacqueline Oxenberg

Additional information is available at the end of the chapter

http://dx.doi.org/10.5772/intechopen.78757

Abstract

While surgery plays a major role in the treatment and potential cure of esophageal cancer, esophagectomy continues to have a significant amount of morbidity compared to other surgical oncology procedures. Efforts to improve morbidity and mortality from esophagectomy include the Consensus Guidelines for Complications from Esophagectomies, Enhanced Recovery after Surgery protocols as well as others. Although we strive to improve morbidity and mortality after these surgeries, adverse events still occur. They affect not only patient quality of life and increase cost of care for esophageal cancer but also have a negative impact on overall cancer survival. This chapter reviews the prevention of adverse outcomes from esophagectomies as well as discusses the management of many complications that may occur more common to the operation.

Keywords: esophagectomy complications, prevention of esophagectomy complications, management of esophagectomy complications

1. Introduction

Adverse events from esophagectomies directly impact patient quality of life, cancer recurrence/survival, hospital costs and resources, as well as require a great deal of energy from those managing them [1, 2]. Prevention of surgical complications is of utmost importance; however, adverse events from this major surgical procedure still occur, even in high-volume centers or experienced hands. Mortality can range from 7 to 9% while morbidity ranges from 17 to 74% [3]. Prevention, early recognition, and adequate management of complications can decrease mortality [4]. While many studies evaluate postoperative morbidity using even randomized methods, randomized studies on the management of postsurgical complications are by nature extremely limited.

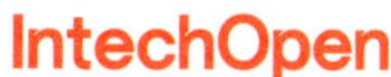

2. Selection of the appropriate patient and surgeon

2.1. The optimal patient

Patient optimization and use of appropriate selection criteria are key to minimizing postoperative morbidity. Unfortunately, those risk factors for the development of esophageal cancer may also put patients at an increased risk for postoperative complications. Risk factors include age, elevated BMI, ECOG score/functional status, dyspnea, diabetes, chronic obstructive pulmonary disease, smoking, alkaline phosphatase level elevations, low serum albumin, and increased complexity score [5–11]. However, age and performance status continue to be the most commonly reported. Neoadjuvant treatments have not been consistently proven to be a risk factor. While fibrosis often occurs after chemoradiation, potentially making surgical resection more difficult, data showing optimal timing to surgery after neoadjuvant chemoradiation and its affect on postoperative morbidity are mixed [12].

2.2. How to optimize the patient

Malnutrition has been reported in 57–80% of patients with esophageal cancer [13, 14]. Many factors can be attributed to malnutrition prior to surgery and include patient factors, chemotherapy, radiation therapy, and tumor-related causes [15]. It is important to recognize that even obese patients can suffer from malnutrition. While laboratory values and anthropometric measurements can be useful, their values can vary and therefore may not be clinically relevant. Therefore, a weight loss of greater than 10% for 6 months or 5% for 1 month is considered malnourished [16].

For the malnourished patient, preoperative optimization of nutrition through the advice of a dietician is key, but other measures should be considered as well if a patient is unable to tolerate at least 50–75% of their caloric needs [15]. The preferred intervention should be handled in a multidisciplinary setting and be initiated as early as possible. This decreases the amount of weight loss, increases chances of completion of neoadjuvant therapies, and decreases hospital admissions [17].

Recommendations to maximize oral nutrition intake include dividing daily oral intake into five to six small meals where the patient is given enough time to eat, eating only foods with a high nutritional content, paying attention to presentation and preparation of meals to make food as desirable as possible, enriching meals and drinks and taking advantage of those days where the patient feels like eating, modifying the consistency of foods to ease swallowing, preventing fatigue, decreasing the risk of aspiration, eating non-irritating soft and smooth foods at room temperature and maintaining oral hygiene for those with mucositis [15]. Patients should also be advised to supplement meals with dietary supplements. The preoperative intake of combined "immunonutrition" products consisting of arginine, glutamine, polyunsaturated omega-3 fatty acids, nucleotides, and antioxidant micronutrients has been shown to decrease postoperative infectious complications and length of hospital stay [15, 18, 19].

For those unable to tolerate adequate nutrition, even with optimization and supplementation, other interventions are needed. These include either stent placement or percutaneous, endoscopic, or surgical placement of feeding gastrostomy or jejunostomy tubes. Esophageal stent placement has the benefit of being placed during endoscopic ultrasound, a common staging procedure. While it may improve dysphagia in the neoadjuvant setting, chest pain can occur and stent migration can be seen in up to 46% of patients [20]. although stent migration can be problematic, it is often a sign of tumor response to neoadjuvant therapy, and therefore the stent may not always need to be replaced. Other reported complications of stent placement in the neoadjuvant setting include perforation, mediastinitis, bowel perforation from migration, tracheo-esophageal fistula, and bleeding [21].

Jejunostomy and gastrostomy tube placement have been proven safe and effective for perioperative nutrition. These can be placed in the laparoscopic, open, endoscopic, or even percutaneous settings. Endoscopic placement may be difficult if a patient has a severe malignant stricture/obstruction, which is often the case when a patient is suffering from severe malnutrition and unable to pass food or liquids through the site of tumor. Gastrostomy tubes have the advantage of bolus feeding, which may improve quality of life. While gastrostomy tube placement has been proven to be safe without increasing the risk of postoperative morbidity, jejunostomy tube placement is often preferred given the stomach is the preferred organ for a neo-esophagus. Jejunostomy tubes are often placed at the time of esophagectomy as well for supportive care. However, some data support that the placement of jejunostomy tubes during esophagectomy is not always necessary [22–24]. Unfortunately, tube feeds cannot be given in boluses with jejunostomy tubes, which, if occurs, can lead to diarrhea and further dehydration. Patients therefore require an ongoing pump connection for feedings.

Smoking cessation is crucial to improving morbidity from esophagectomy. This may be most beneficial if performed greater than 90 days before surgery [25]. Active smoking has also been shown to increase recurrence rates of cancer after esophagectomy [26]. Therefore, smoking cessation counseling and supportive programs are necessary when patients are being assessed for esophagectomy.

2.3. The optimal surgeon/hospital

When deciding the optimal surgeon, it is important to understand that outcomes depend on two major factors: experience and resources. It is well known that with increasing numbers of esophagectomies performed, postoperative morbidity and mortality are improved. In addition, long-term survival can also improve [27]. While data show improved outcomes at higher volume centers, this is inconsistent and may depend further on individual surgeon volumes and hospital resources [28]. Begg et al. described low-volume hospitals as 1–5 esophagectomies/year, medium volume 6–11 esophagectomies/year, and high-volume centers as those performing >11 esophagectomies/year, with an improved mortality with increasing hospital volumes [29]. Later, Birkmeyer et al. divided hospital volumes to <2 esophagectomies/year as low-volume and high-volume centers as >19 esophagectomies/year [30]. The 2003 Leapfrog Group recommended 13 esophagectomies/year as a minimum volume standard [31]. However, esophagectomies at mid-volume centers can also be safely performed, especially with a two-surgeon approach [32]. Hospital type may also be important where improved reoperation rates and mortality are seen when surgery is performed at University centers or institutions centralizing esophageal cancer care [33–35].

Early recognition and treatment of complications appears to be just as important as prevention to improve mortality [36]. The recognition of postoperative problems improves with experience, making hospital volumes as well as surgeon volumes important. With morbidity rates being high, early intervention is of utmost importance to prevent further adverse outcomes or even death. In fact, even in low-volume hospitals, mortality may remain low if adequate resources are available [28, 37]. Therefore, these surgeries should only be performed at institutions well equipped to handle the possible complications [38–40]. Ancillary departments that should be available in the postoperative care may include gastroenterology, interventional radiology, cardiology, an astute critical care team, and others. Resources readily available and proven to improve complications also include nurse-to-patient ratios, where the incidence of pulmonary and infectious complications was shown to be increased when nurses had more than two patients [41].

2.4. Optimal surgical approach

Tumor location as well as surgeon experience often dictates the type of surgery performed. Multiple accepted operative approaches to esophageal carcinoma include Ivor Lewis esophagogastrectomy, McKeown esophagogastrectomy, transhiatal esophagogastrectomy, and left transthoracic or thoracoabdominal approaches. Minimally invasive techniques include laparoscopic and robotic esophagectomies. While minimally invasive esophagectomies have been shown to be safe and effective with equivalent oncologic outcomes, robotic, rather than laparoscopic approaches are becoming common [42–44]. However, one should be aware that there is a learning curve when a surgeon is transitioning to minimally invasive esophagectomies [45]. Transthoracic esophagectomies include the Ivor Lewis esophagogastrectomy and the McKeown esophagogastrectomy. Morbidity varies on the location of the anastomosis and if the transthoracic approach was used. While the transthoracic approach may have an increased morbidity, it does allow for extended lymphadenectomies to be performed, possibly increasing long-term survival [10, 46] .

3. Prevention and management of complications

The Esophagectomy Complications Consensus Group (ECCG) is a group of 21 high-volume surgeons from 14 countries that compiled a complete list of complications from esophagectomies [3]. These adverse events are separated into pulmonary, cardiac, gastrointestinal, urologic, thromboembolic, neurologic/psychiatric, infectious, wound/diaphragm, and others. They also aimed to standardize the definitions and reporting of complications since reported literature varied depending on adverse reactions and even mortality definitions. These definitions were defined for anastomotic leak, conduit necrosis, chyle leak and vocal cord injury/palsy. Given the large number of possible complications, this chapter reviews those more common or even specific to esophagectomy.

3.1. Atrial fibrillation

Atrial fibrillation can occur in over 20% of patients undergoing esophagectomy, particularly when the transthoracic approach is used [47, 48]. Its occurrence unfortunately can result in hemodynamic instability as well as put patients at an increased risk for stroke. Atrial Fibrillation may also be an early warning sign for morbidity, especially anastomotic leak [49]. The mechanism and pathophysiology of postoperative atrial fibrillation is incompletely understood, although we know predisposing factors include advanced age, coronary artery disease, heart failure, hypertension, mitral valve disease, and previous history of atrial fibrillation [50]. One randomized, controlled trial showed that the preoperative use of amiodarone via IV infusion significantly reduced the incidence of atrial fibrillation; however, no differences were seen in median hospital stay, ICU stay, or adverse events [51]. In a study evaluating amiodarone administration through the jejunostomy tube postoperatively, there was only a trend towards lower occurrence and a shorter length of stay [52]. Beta-blockers should be continued for the prevention of atrial fibrillation as well if a patient is already taking them, but may require a reduced dose for the prevention of hypotension, especially with epidural anesthesia. Calcium channel blockers, particularly diltiazem, can also be used for the prevention of atrial fibrillation and may have less effect on blood pressure than other calcium channel blockers or beta-blockers [53]. If atrial fibrillation occurs, amiodarone, calcium channel blockers, and beta-blockers are all treatments to be considered, depending on the patient's hemodynamics.

3.2. Respiratory failure/pneumonia/prolonged ventilation

Respiratory complications in patients undergoing esophagectomy can be problematic and are often causes of mortality. When patients need to be reintubated, many require bag ventilation or positive pressure prior to intubation, which may cause insufflation of the esophagus and stomach, placing pressure on the anastomosis or staple lines. For that reason, CPAP is often avoided as well. Direct airway visualization during reintubation is also important to prevent mechanical injury in case the esophagus is intubated rather than the trachea, especially if a cervical anastomosis is performed.

Pneumonia has been shown to significantly increase mortality compared to other complications, even anastomotic leak [6, 8]. Unfortunately, it can also be the most common postoperative complication and cause for respiratory failure and prolonged ventilation [7]. The American Thoracic Society and American Infections Diseases Society define pneumonia into hospital-acquired pneumonia (HAP), ventilator-associated pneumonia (VAP), and health-care-associated pneumonia (HCAP) [54]. The revised Uniform Pneumonia Score aims to define pneumonia occurring after esophagectomies and includes temperature, leukocyte count, and pulmonary radiographic findings [55]. Prevention, early recognition, and treatment as well as correction of causes are key.

Aspiration is a major cause of pneumonia. This occurs more often with a cervical anastomosis, especially with recurrent laryngeal nerve injury. Recurrent laryngeal nerve palsy can occur secondary to stretching, thermal injury, or even compression. If occurs, patients may suffer from hoarseness as well as pulmonary complications such as dyspnea and aspiration, which puts them at an increased risk for pneumonia and reintubation/prolonged ventilation. However, recurrent laryngeal nerve injury may not always present as obvious hoarseness, as we know from thyroid surgery data, and therefore its occurrence may be underreported. The ECCG defines vocal cord injury/palsy as a vocal cord dysfunction postresection where confirmation and assessment are achieved by direct examination [3]. There are three types of injuries/palsies that are each further separated into unilateral (A) and bilateral (B): Type 1 includes a transient injury requiring no therapy, where only dietary modifications are needed; Type 2 is an injury requiring elective surgical procedures such as thyroplasty or medialization procedures; Type 3 is an injury requiring acute surgical intervention due to aspiration or other respiratory issues that include thyroplasty or medialization procedures. Injury to the left recurrent laryngeal nerve is most common and is mainly associated with esophagectomies that include cervical anastomoses or dissections, McKeown-type operations. Therefore, prevention may include performing thoracic anastomoses or careful dissection and prevention of injury from the above causes. The early recognition of injury and treatment (which may include medialization of the vocal fold) may prevent aspiration and pneumonia and therefore may be of benefit early in the postoperative course [56, 57].

Other causes of respiratory failure or shortness of breath can include ARDS, cardiac causes, pleural effusions, pneumothorax, phrenic nerve injury, or fistula. Other infections can put patients at risk for ARDS (acute respiratory distress syndrome), and cardiac causes may also result in respiratory failure and need for reintubation. If ARDS occurs, the cause should be evaluated, including examining for other infections (urine, leak, etc.). If cardiac in nature, most commonly secondary to atrial fibrillation, heart rate control is usually necessary to alleviate symptoms. Pleural effusions and pneumothorax are common and can be managed with chest tube placement or percutaneous radiologic drainage, depending on the size of the effusion or pneumothorax. If effusions occur simultaneously with anastomotic leak, adequate drainage should be performed to prevent empyema and life-threatening mediastinitis. While phrenic nerve injury is rare, immediate surgical intervention is not always needed. However, patients may require tracheostomy placement for pulmonary conditioning. It is also important to remember that patients are at an increased risk for deep vein thrombosis and even pulmonary embolism. This may occur prior to or even after esophagectomy. Perioperative prophylactic anticoagulation should be administered in the perioperative setting to prevent deep vein thrombosis/pulmonary embolism. Tracheoesophageal fistula should also be considered, especially later in the recovery period or in a complicated postoperative recovery setting.

Impaired lung function is a significant risk factor for pulmonary complications [8]. With preoperative chemoradiation, pneumonitis can occur, making patients at an increased risk for postoperative respiratory failure and pneumonia [8]. While some degree of inflammation is often seen in preoperative imaging, assuring patient lung function has not decompensated is prudent. This can often cause delays in surgery; however, allowing the recovery of lung function may improve postoperative pulmonary failure.

Consistent with the recommendations of the Enhanced Recovery After Surgery pathways, intravenous fluid administration should be minimized to improve time to return of bowel function and decrease the length of hospital stay. Excessive fluid administration/fluid overload should also be considered in all patients with acute respiratory failure since the administration of diuretics may quickly improve symptoms.

3.3. *Anastomotic leak/conduit necrosis*

Anastomotic leak after esophagectomy can be difficult to manage and has a major impact on patient quality of life as well as may affect long-term survival [58, 59]. Incidence varies from 5.7 to 14.3% with a higher incidence in cervical anastomoses versus thoracic [60]. The International Study Group for Rectal Cancer proposed the verbiage of anastomotic leak as, "A defect of the integrity in a surgical joint between two hollow viscera with communication between the intraluminal and extraluminal compartments," which was later validated and expanded to the entire gastrointestinal tract [61]. Lerut et al. with the Surgery Infection Study Group defined anastomotic leak severity as Type 1, a radiological leak without any clinical findings; Type 2 with minor clinical findings of local inflammation (cervical wound) or X-ray showed suppressed leak (thoracic anastomosis); Type 3, a major clinical leak with severe disruption and sepsis; Type 4, conduit necrosis seen by endoscopic confirmation [62]. The Early Complications Consensus Group (ECCG) defined anastomotic leak as a full-thickness GI defect involving esophagus, anastomosis, staple line, or conduit, irrespective of the presentation of the method of identification [3]. Type 1 includes a local defect requiring no change in therapy or treated medically or with dietary modification. Type 2 is a localized defect requiring interventional but not surgical therapy (interventional radiology drainage, stent or bedside opening and packing of incision). Type 3 is a localized defect requiring surgical therapy.

Many patient factors as well as peri- and intraoperative factors can contribute to anastomotic leak. Patients at an increased risk for anastomotic leak include those with increased comorbidities, advanced pathologic stage, prior esophagogastric surgeries, and active smoking [63]. Patient factors can include preoperative malnutrition, diabetes, prolonged hospitalization, hypotension, hypoxemia, preoperative chemotherapy, preoperative chemoradiation, and age. Technical factors also impacting the rate of anastomotic leak include the location of the anastomosis, surgery type, tension on the anastomosis, the type of anastomosis (hand sewn vs. stapled), arterial and venous insufficiency, excessive bleeding, and surgeon experience. While leak incidence may be higher in a single-layer anastomosis, the incidence of stricture may be higher in a double-layer anastomosis [64–66]. While data are mixed, the incidence of leak and stricture may also be lower with a stapled anastomosis [67, 68]. Postoperative factors may include gastric distention, external compression, infection, re-exploration for bleeding, prolonged mechanical ventilation, and continued hypoxemia and hypotension [69]. Technical considerations to decrease the rate of anastomotic leak may include anastomotic support with omentum, pleura, pericardium, and fat tissue. Prospective randomized studies have shown that omental wrapping of the anastomosis may decrease the rate of leak or even stricture [70, 71].

Diagnosis can be made by clinical suspicion if a patient presents with fevers, leukocytosis, empyema, pleural effusion, pneumomediastinum, increased drainage from the chest tube (bile or other gastric contents), the presence of enteric bacteria or bacterial culture or tachycardia. The early detection of anastomotic leaks may also include CRP/ESR elevation, an increase in procalcitonin level, and leukocytosis extending past the second and fifth postoperative days, respectively [72, 73]. While contrast esophagogram can be performed to determine subclinical leaks, caution is advised given the risks of aspiration [4, 74]. A barium swallow can be performed to detect an anastomotic leak; however, its sensitivity can be relatively low and may often be performed too early to detect [75, 76]. The oral intake of methylene blue may be used given it is otherwise nontoxic. CT scan with oral contrast may also be helpful and show contrast extravasation as well as concerning areas for infection.

The etiology of the leak is vital to ascertain where patients with conduit tip necrosis or complete conduit ischemia may require different interventions. This often requires direct visualization with EGD for conduit evaluation as well as evaluation of the defect size. The ECCG defines conduit necrosis into three types, with recommendations for specific treatments: Type 1 includes a focal conduit necrosis that is identified endoscopically, requiring only additional monitoring or nonsurgical therapy; Type 2 includes focal conduit necrosis that is identified endoscopically and is not associated with free anastomotic or conduit leak. Surgical therapy not involving esophageal diversion is performed; Type 3 includes extensive conduit necrosis that is treated with conduit resection and diversion [3].

If a leak occurs, source control with drain placement with or without operative intervention remains key to preventing mortality. For this reason, intraoperative drain placement for detection and source control is common. Management often is determined by anastomotic location; however, mediastinitis can occur with both intrathoracic and cervical anastomoses, a possibly fatal diagnosis for which requires close monitoring and rapid evaluation and treatment. Turkyilmaz et al. created algorithms to help guide treatment for anastomotic leak. For cervical anastomoses, a limited leak that is clinically occult may be managed with antibiotics, dressing changes, and cleansing with oral isotonic fluid. If there is a clinically prominent cervical leak, antibiotics, opening of the cervical wound, drain placement, nasogastric decompression, nutritional support, and cleaning are typically needed. For cervical anastomotic leaks that have intrathoracic complications and clinical sepsis failing to improve, drain placement, stent placement, decortication, resection/diversion or resection/colonic interposition may be needed. For thoracic anastomoses, if a contained leak with less than 30% disruption, injection with fibrin glue, endoclips, or stents can be used for management. However, if the defect is larger, drainage and esophageal stent placement can be performed followed by surgery if stent placement and drainage are unsuccessful (can include primary or supporting tissue repair). However, if the anastomosis has a greater than 70% disruption, surgery including drainage and primary repair should be performed first with esophageal diversion with possible colonic interposition if unable to be performed [69].

With the use of self-expanding metal stents, endoscopic management alone has become possible for anastomotic leaks/disruptions. Covered stents can be placed to control the leak, preventing further seeding into the mediastinum for both cervical and thoracic anastomoses. If well controlled, oral intake may also be safe. However, stent migration can occur, requiring retrieval and replacement [77]. Stent use may be limited in large defects (which may occur from conduit necrosis or staple line disruption). It is also important to understand that lumen caliber differences between the esophagus and gastric conduit can result in the reflux of gastric contents around the distal aspect of a stent. This unfortunately may not be seen with an esophagogram, but rather be noticed with other imaging such as CT after the reflux of contrast and gastric contents occur and may be delayed. Therefore, other options for control have emerged including endoscopic vacuum-assisted closure devices and may even be more effective than stent placement [78–81].

3.4. Fistula

In addition to source control, the awareness and prevention of esophago/gastrotracheal fistula is also necessary. This can occur from infection itself or even the erosion of foreign material (stent, staples, etc.) into the trachea. One should be suspicious in patients with frequent uncontrolled coughing, especially after swallowing, or "Ono's sign" [82]. Workup and diagnosis can include an upper gastrointestinal X-ray with oral contrast or even direct visualization with esophagoscopy or bronchoscopy. Prevention may include a pleural wrap around the anastomosis at the time of original operation or even at the time of reoperation if a leak occurs and anastomotic repair is possible. If reoperation is not performed, stent placement may help control symptoms and healing [83]. However, distal feeding tube placement and resection may be needed. Treatment is necessary to prevent recurring pneumonia.

3.5. Delayed gastric emptying

Delayed or inappropriate gastric emptying can occur secondary to the disruption of vagal nerve complexes to the stomach. This can result in delayed emptying of the stomach, which affects not only patient quality of life and inability to obtain oral nutrition but also can put patients at an increased risk for reflux of gastric contents and even aspiration. The most common options for the management of the pylorus include pyloromyotomy, pyloroplasty, intra-pyloric botulinum toxin injection as well as no intervention. While one multicenter study showed no significant difference between pyloroplasty, botulinum toxin-injection, and no pyloric treatment, one study did show that intra-pyloric botulinum toxin can increase the risk of postoperative reflux and increase the use of promotility agents and endoscopic interventions [84, 85]. While delayed gastric emptying can occur anywhere from 10 to 50%, it also can be successfully managed with prokinetic agents (75%) and endoscopic dilation [86].

3.6. Chyle leak/chylothorax

With the thoracic duct being the largest lymphatic vessel in the body as well as being located in the chest, posterior to the esophagus, injury can occur. Its location, however, often varies. The incidence of chyle leak is rather low (1–4%); however, when it occurs, it can be very problematic [87]. Chyle contains triglycerides in the form of chylomicrons as well as lymphocytes. Chyle leaks can result in malnutrition (with continued protein loss), immune compromise, hypovolemia, electrolyte abnormalities, hypoalbuminemia, lymphopenia, and infection [88]. The ECCG defines a chyle leak into three different types, where output <1 L/day is further classified as "A," and "B" is further classified as >1 L/day [3]. Type 1 leaks can be managed with enteric dietary modifications alone. Type 2 can be managed with total parenteral nutrition. Type 3 requires management with interventional or surgical therapy.

Following esophagectomy, drainage from a chest tube of >500 mL/day is suggestive of a chyle leak; however, the measurement of chylomicrons or triglycerides is most commonly utilized [89]. A measurement of >4% chylomicrons or fluid containing >100–110 mg/dL of triglycerides is typically considered indicative of a chyle leak. Since a chyle leak may present with increased serous or even serosanguinous drainage while fasting, a clinical diagnosis can be made by the oral intake of cream followed by milky drainage from the chest tube/drains.

Prevention unfortunately is difficult. Selective en masse ligation has been shown to reduce the rate of chylothorax [90]. Also, the preoperative oral administration of cream may help identify the thoracic duct to aid in the prevention of its injury or to identify the thoracic duct for prophylactic ligation [91]. The initial management of a chyle leak usually includes drainage as well as TPN and bowel rest. Decreasing oral or enteral fat intake decreases the flow of chyle through the leak, possibly allowing spontaneous closure [92]. Long chain fatty acids should be avoided with diets supported by high percentages of medium-chain triglycerides since they are typically absorbed directly into intestinal cells, bypassing the thoracic duct [87]. If conservative management is not successful, surgical intervention may be necessary, especially if the fistula is of high output. Aggressive surgical intervention should be performed if chyle output is >1.5 L/day for >5–7 days [93]. Surgical intervention includes thoracotomy or thoracoscopic thoracic duct ligation on the side of the chylothorax. This is usually assisted by the preoperative administration of cream or lipophilic dye to help identify the thoracic duct. If the leak can be localized, this may be controlled with clips or suture; however, if the leak is unclear, ligation of the thoracic duct just cephalad to the aortic hiatus is recommended [94–96]. Pleurodesis can also be performed at the time of ligation as well.

Radiologic-guided/percutaneous embolization is becoming more popular, especially for patients who are poor operative candidates. This includes lymphangiography followed by transabdominal percutaneous needle cannulation, although a retrograde subclavian vein approach can be used [97, 98]. Once the cisterna chyli is canalized, a catheter is advanced into the thoracic duct and contrast used to identify the leak. Embolization can then be performed. Since surgical intervention to ligate the thoracic duct using thoracoscopy or a thoracotomy can result in increased morbidity and mortality, thoracic duct embolization has become increasingly more popular when conservative management fails.

Author details

Jacqueline Oxenberg

Address all correspondence to: jcoxenberg@geisinger.edu

Geisinger Wyoming Valley, Wilkes-Barre, PA, USA

References

[1] Kataoka K, Takeuchi H, Mizusawa J, et al. Prognostic impact of postoperative morbidity after esophagectomy for esophageal cancer: Exploratory analysis of JCOG9907. Annals of Surgery. 2017;**265**(6):1152-1157. DOI: 10.1097/SLA.0000000000001828

[2] Lerut T, Moons J, Coosemans W, et al. Postoperative complications after transthoracic esophagectomy for cancer of the esophagus and gastroesophageal junction are correlated with early cancer recurrence: Role of systematic grading of complications using the modified clavien classification. Annals of Surgery. 2009;**250**(5):798-806. DOI: 10.1097/SLA.0b013e3181bdd5a8

[3] Low DE, Alderson D, Cecconello I, et al. International consensus on standardization of data collection for complications associated with esophagectomy: Esophagectomy complications consensus group (ECCG). Annals of Surgery. 2015;**262**(2):286-294. DOI: 10.1097/SLA.0000000000001098

[4] Griffin SM, Lamb PJ, Dresner SM, Richardson DL, Hayes N. Diagnosis and management of a mediastinal leak following radical oesophagectomy. The British Journal of Surgery. 2001;**88**(10):1346-1351. DOI: 10.1046/j.0007-1323.2001.01918.x

[5] Law S, Wong K, Kwok K, Chu K, Wong J. Predictive factors for postoperative pulmonary complications and mortality after esophagectomy for cancer. Annals of Surgery. 2004;**240**(5):791-800. DOI: 10.1097/01.sla.0000143123.24556.1c

[6] Atkins BZ, Shah AS, Hutcheson KA, et al. Reducing hospital morbidity and mortality following esophagectomy. The Annals of Thoracic Surgery. 2004;**78**(4):1170-1176. DOI: 10.1016/j.athoracsur.2004.02.034

[7] Bailey SH, Bull DA, Harpole DH, et al. Outcomes after esophagectomy: A ten-year prospective cohort. The Annals of Thoracic Surgery. 2003;**75**(1):217-222. DOI: 10.1016/S0003-4975(02)04368-0

[8] Avendano CE, Flume PA, Silvestri GA, King LB, Reed CE. Pulmonary complications after esophagectomy. The Annals of Thoracic Surgery. 2002;**73**(3):922-926. DOI: 10.1016/S0003-4975(01)03584-6

[9] Kinugasa S, Tachibana M, Yoshimura H, et al. Postoperative pulmonary complications are associated with worse short- and long-term outcomes after extended esophagectomy. Journal of Surgical Oncology. 2004;**88**(2):71-77. DOI: 10.1002/jso.20137

[10] Raymond DP, Seder CW, Wright CD, et al. Predictors of major morbidity or mortality after resection for esophageal cancer: A society of thoracic surgeons general thoracic surgery database risk adjustment model. The Annals of Thoracic Surgery. 2016;**102**(1):207-214. DOI: 10.1016/j.athoracsur.2016.04.055

[11] Ferguson MK, Martin TR, Reeder LB, Olak J. Mortality after esophagectomy: Risk factor analysis. World Journal of Surgery. 1997;**21**(6):599-604. DOI: 10.1007/s002689900279

[12] Kim JY, Correa AM, Vaporciyan AA, et al. Does the timing of esophagectomy after chemoradiation affect outcome? The Annals of Thoracic Surgery. 2012;**93**(1):207-212; discussion 212-3. DOI: 10.1016/j.athoracsur.2011.05.021

[13] Daly JM, Fry WA, Little AG, et al. Esophageal cancer: Results of American college of surgeons patient care evaluation study. Journal of the American College of Surgeons. 2000;**190**(5):562-573

[14] Dewys WD, Begg C, Lavin PT, et al. Prognostic effect of weight loss prior to chemotherapy in cancer patients. Eastern cooperative oncology group. The American Journal of Medicine. 1980;**69**(4):491-497

[15] Mariette C, De Botton M, Piessen G. Surgery in esophageal and gastric cancer patients: What is the role for nutrition support in your daily practice? Annals of Surgical Oncology. 2012;**19**(7):2128-2134. DOI: 10.1245/s10434-012-2225-6

[16] Nitenberg G, Raynard B. Nutritional support of the cancer patient: Issues and dilemmas. Critical Reviews in Oncology/Hematology. 2000;**34**(3):137-168. DOI: 10.1016/S1040-8428(00)00048-2

[17] Odelli C, Burgess D, Bateman L, et al. Nutrition support improves patient outcomes, treatment tolerance and admission characteristics in oesophageal cancer. Clinical Oncology. 2005;**17**(8):639-645. DOI: 10.1016/j.clon.2005.03.015

[18] Beale RJ, Bryg DJ, Bihari DJ. Immunonutrition in the critically ill: A systematic review of clinical outcome. Critical Care Medicine. 1999;**27**(12):2799-2805. DOI: 10.1097/00003246-199912000-00032

[19] Heys SD, Walker LG, Smith I, Eremin O. Enteral nutritional supplementation with key nutrients in patients with critical illness and caner: A meta-analysis of randomized controlled clinical trials. Nutrition Clinique et Metabolisme. 2000;**14**(1):62-63

[20] Adler DG, Fang J, Wong R, Wills J, Hilden K. Placement of polyflex stents in patients with locally advanced esophageal cancer is safe and improves dysphagia during neoadjuvant therapy. Gastrointestinal Endoscopy. 2009;**70**(4):614-619. DOI: 10.1016/j.gie.2009.01.026

[21] Langer FB, Schoppmann SF, Prager G, et al. Temporary placement of self-expanding oesophageal stents as bridging for neo-adjuvant therapy. Annals of Surgical Oncology. 2010;**17**(2):470-475. DOI: 10.1245/s10434-009-0760-6

[22] Srinathan SK, Hamin T, Walter S, Tan AL, Unruh HW, Guyatt G. Jejunostomy tube feeding in patients undergoing esophagectomy. Canadian Journal of Surgery. 2013;**56**(6):409-414. DOI: 10.1503/cjs.008612

[23] Fenton JR, Bergeron EJ, Coello M, Welsh RJ, Chmielewski GW. Feeding jejunostomy tubes placed during esophagectomy: Are they necessary? The Annals of Thoracic Surgery. 2011;**92**(2):504-11; discussion 511-2. DOI: 10.1016/j.athoracsur.2011.03.101

[24] Weijs TJ, van Eden HWJ, Ruurda JP, et al. Routine jejunostomy tube feeding following esophagectomy. Journal of Thoracic Disease. 2017;**9**:S851-S860. DOI: 10.21037/jtd.2017.06.73

[25] Yoshida N, Baba Y, Hiyoshi Y, et al. Duration of smoking cessation and postoperative morbidity after esophagectomy for esophageal cancer: How long should patients stop smoking before surgery? World Journal of Surgery. 2016;**40**(1):142-147. DOI: 10.1007/s00268-015-3236-9

[26] Mantziari S, Allemann P, Winiker M, Demartines N, Schäfer M. Locoregional tumor extension and preoperative smoking are significant risk factors for early recurrence after esophagectomy for cancer. World Journal of Surgery. 2017;**42**(7):2209-2217. DOI: 10.1007/s00268-017-4422-8

[27] Brusselaers N, Mattsson F, Lagergren J. Hospital and surgeon volume in relation to long-term survival after oesophagectomy: Systematic review and meta-analysis. Gut. 2014;**63**(9):1393-1400. DOI: 10.1136/gutjnl-2013-306074

[28] Varghese TK, Wood DE, Farjah F, et al. Variation in esophagectomy outcomes in hospitals meeting leapfrog volume outcome standards. The Annals of Thoracic Surgery. 2011;**91**(4):1003-1009. DOI: 10.1016/j.athoracsur.2010.11.006

[29] Begg CB, Cramer LD, Hoskins WJ, Brennan MF. Impact of hospital volume on operative mortality for major cancer surgery. Journal of the American Medical Association. 1998;**280**(20):1747-1751

[30] Birkmeyer JD, Lucas FL, Wennberg DE. Potential benefits of regionalizing major surgery in medicare patients. Effective Clinical Practice. 1999;**2**(6):277-283

[31] Birkmeyer JD, Dimick JB. Potential benefits of the new leapfrog standards: Effect of process and outcomes measures. Surgery. 2004;**135**(6):569-575. DOI: 10.1016/j.surg.2004.03.004

[32] McCahill LE, May M, Morrow JB, et al. Esophagectomy outcomes at a mid-volume cancer center utilizing prospective multidisciplinary care and a 2-surgeon team approach. American Journal of Surgery. 2014;**207**(3):380-386. DOI: 10.1016/j.amjsurg.2013.09.013

[33] Kauppila JH, Wahlin K, Lagergren P, Lagergren J. University hospital status and surgeon volume and risk of reoperation following surgery for esophageal cancer. European Journal of Surgical Oncology. 2018;**44**(5):632-637. DOI: 10.1016/j.ejso.2018.02.212

[34] Varagunam M, Hardwick R, Riley S, Chadwick G, Cromwell DA, Groene O. Changes in volume, clinical practice and outcome after reorganisation of oesophago-gastric cancer care in England: A longitudinal observational study. European Journal of Surgical Oncology. 2018;**44**(4):524-531. DOI: 10.1016/j.ejso.2018.01.001

[35] Hummel R, Ha NH, Lord A, Trochsler MI, Maddern G, Kanhere H. Centralisation of oesophagectomy in Australia: Is only caseload critical? Australian Health Review. 2017. DOI: 10.1071/AH17095

[36] Michael Griffin S, Shaw IH, Dresner SM. Early complications after ivorlewis subtotal esophagectomy with two-field lymphadenectomy: Risk factors and management. Journal of the American College of Surgeons. 2002;**194**(3):285-297. DOI: 10.1016/S1072-7515(01)01177-2

[37] Funk LM, Gawande AA, Semel ME, et al. Esophagectomy outcomes at low-volume hospitals: The association between systems characteristics and mortality. Annals of Surgery. 2011;**253**(5):912-917. DOI: 10.1097/SLA.0b013e318213862f

[38] Dudley RA, Johansen KL, Brand R, Rennie DJ, Milstein A. Selective referral to high-volume hospitals: Estimating potentially avoidable deaths. Journal of the American Medical Association. 2000;**283**(9):1159-1166

[39] Birkmeyer JD, Siewers AE, Finlayson EVA, et al. Hospital volume and surgical mortality in the United States. New England Journal of Medicine. 2002;**346**(15):1128-1137. DOI: 10.1056/NEJMsa012337

[40] Halm EA, Lee C, Chassin MR. Is volume related to outcome in health care? A systematic review and methodologic critique of the literature. Annals of Internal Medicine. 2002;**137**(6):511-520

[41] Amaravadi RK, Dimick JB, Pronovost PJ, Lipsett PA. ICU nurse-to-patient ratio is associated with complications and resource use after esophagectomy. Intensive Care Medicine. 2000;**26**(12):1857-1862. DOI: 10.1007/s001340000720

[42] Pennathur A, Farkas A, Krasinskas AM, et al. Esophagectomy for T1 esophageal cancer: Outcomes in 100 patients and implications for endoscopic therapy. The Annals of Thoracic Surgery. 2009;**87**(4):1048-1055. DOI: 10.1016/j.athoracsur.2008.12.060

[43] Luketich JD, Pennathur A, Awais O, et al. Outcomes after minimally invasive esophagectomy: Review of over 1000 patients. Annals of Surgery. 2012;**256**(1):95-103. DOI: 10.1097/SLA.0b013e3182590603

[44] Luketich JD, Pennathur A, Franchetti Y, et al. Minimally invasive esophagectomy: Results of a prospective phase II multicenter trial-the eastern cooperative oncology group (E2202) study. Annals of Surgery. 2015;**261**(4):702-707. DOI: 10.1097/SLA.0000000000000993

[45] Sarkaria IS, Rizk NP, Grosser R, et al. Attaining proficiency in robotic-assisted minimally invasive esophagectomy while maximizing safety during procedure development. Innovations Technology and Techniques in Cardiothoracic and Vascular Surgery. 2016; **11**(4):268-273. DOI: 10.1097/IMI.0000000000000297

[46] Junginger T, Gockel I, Heckhoff S. A comparison of transhiatal and transthoracic resections on the prognosis in patients with squamous cell carcinoma of the esophagus. European Journal of Surgical Oncology. 2006;**32**(7):749-755. DOI: 10.1016/j.ejso.2006.03.048

[47] Stawicki SPA, Prosciak MP, Gerlach AT, et al. Atrial fibrillation after esophagectomy: An indicator of postoperative morbidity. General Thoracic and Cardiovascular Surgery. 2011;**59**(6):399-405. DOI: 10.1007/s11748-010-0713-9

[48] Lohani KR, Nandipati KC, Rollins SE, et al. Transthoracic approach is associated with increased incidence of atrial fibrillation after esophageal resection. Surgical Endoscopy. 2015;**29**(7):2039-2045. DOI: 10.1007/s00464-014-3908-9

[49] Seesing MFJ, Scheijmans JCG, Borggreve AS, van Hillegersberg R, Ruurda JP. The predictive value of new-onset atrial fibrillation on postoperative morbidity after esophagectomy. Diseases of the Esophagus. 2018. DOI: 10.1093/dote/doy028

[50] Turagam MK, Downey FX, Kress DC, Sra J, Tajik AJ, Jahangir A. Pharmacological strategies for prevention of postoperative atrial fibrillation. Expert Review of Clinical Pharmacology. 2015;**8**(2):233-250. DOI: 10.1586/17512433.2015.1018182

[51] Tisdale JE, Wroblewski HA, Wall DS, et al. A randomized, controlled study of amiodarone for prevention of atrial fibrillation after transthoracic esophagectomy. The Journal of Thoracic and Cardiovascular Surgery. 2010;**140**(1):45-51. DOI: 10.1016/j.jtcvs.2010.01.026

[52] Fabian T, Rassias DJ, Daneshmand MA, Ilves R. Amiodarone for atrial fibrillation prophylaxis in patients undergoing esophagectomy. Chest. 2004;**126**(4):800S

[53] Fernando HC, Jaklitsch MT, Walsh GL, et al. The society of thoracic surgeons practice guideline on the prophylaxis and management of atrial fibrillation associated with

general thoracic surgery: Executive summary. The Annals of Thoracic Surgery. 2011; **92**(3):1144-1152. DOI: 10.1016/j.athoracsur.2011.06.104

[54] Kalil AC, Metersky ML, Klompas M, et al. Executive summary: Management of adults with hospital-acquired and ventilator-associated pneumonia: 2016 clinical practice guidelines by the infectious diseases society of America and the American thoracic society. Clinical Infectious Diseases. 2016;**63**(5):575-582. DOI: 10.1093/cid/ciw504

[55] Weijs TJ, Seesing MFJ, van Rossum PSN, et al. Internal and external validation of a multivariable model to define hospital-acquired pneumonia after esophagectomy. Journal of Gastrointestinal Surgery. 2016;**20**(4):680-687. DOI: 10.1007/s11605-016-3083-5

[56] Bhattacharyya N, Batirel H, Swanson SJ. Improved outcomes with early vocal fold medialization for vocal fold paralysis after thoracic surgery. Auris, Nasus, Larynx. 2003;**30**(1):71-75. DOI: 10.1016/S0385-8146(02)00114-1

[57] Scholtemeijer MG, Seesing MFJ, Brenkman HJF, Janssen LM, van Hillegersberg R, Ruurda JP. Recurrent laryngeal nerve injury after esophagectomy for esophageal cancer: Incidence, management, and impact on short- and long-term outcomes. Journal of Thoracic Disease. 2017;**9**(Suppl 8):S868-S878. DOI: 10.21037/jtd.2017.06.92 [doi]

[58] Sierzega M, Kolodziejczyk P, Kulig J. Impact of anastomotic leakage on long-term survival after total gastrectomy for carcinoma of the stomach. The British Journal of Surgery. 2010;**97**(7):1035-1042. DOI: 10.1002/bjs.7038

[59] Rizk NP, Ishwaran H, Rice TW, et al. Optimum lymphadenectomy for esophageal cancer. Annals of Surgery. 2010;**251**(1):46-50. DOI: 10.1097/SLA.0b013e3181b2f6ee

[60] Kassis ES, Kosinski AS, Ross P, Koppes KE, Donahue JM, Daniel VC. Predictors of anastomotic leak after esophagectomy: An analysis of the society of thoracic surgeons general thoracic database. The Annals of Thoracic Surgery. 2013;**96**(6):1919-1926. DOI: 10.1016/j.athoracsur.2013.07.119

[61] Chadi SA, Fingerhut A, Berho M, et al. Emerging trends in the etiology, prevention, and treatment of gastrointestinal anastomotic leakage. Journal of Gastrointestinal Surgery. 2016;**20**(12):2035-2051. DOI: 10.1007/s11605-016-3255-3

[62] Lerut T, Coosemans W, Decker G, De Leyn P, Nafteux P, Van Raemdonck D. Anastomotic complications after esophagectomy. Digestive Surgery. 2002;**19**(2):92-98. DOI: 10.1159/000052018

[63] Cooke DT, Lin GC, Lau CL, et al. Analysis of cervical esophagogastric anastomotic leaks after transhiatal esophagectomy: Risk factors, presentation, and detection. The Annals of Thoracic Surgery. 2009;**88**(1):177-185. DOI: 10.1016/j.athoracsur.2009.03.035

[64] Wilson SE, Stone R, Scully M, Ozeran L, Benfield JR. Modern management of anastomotic leak after esophagogastrectomy. American Journal of Surgery. 1982;**144**(1):95-101. DOI: 10.1016/0002-9610(82)90608-0

[65] Mathisen DJ, Grillo HC, Wilkins EW Jr, Moncure AC, Hilgenberg AD. Transthoracic esophagectomy: A safe approach to carcinoma of the esophagus. The Annals of Thoracic Surgery. 1988;**45**(2):137-143

[66] Postlethwait RW. Complications and deaths after operations for esophageal carcinoma. The Journal of Thoracic and Cardiovascular Surgery. 1983;**85**(6):827-831

[67] Okuyama M, Motoyama S, Suzuki H, Saito R, Maruyama K, Ogawa J. Hand-sewn cervical anastomosis versus stapled intrathoracic anastomosis after esophagectomy for middle or lower thoracic esophageal cancer: A prospective randomized controlled study. Surgery Today. 2007;**37**(11):947-952. DOI: 10.1007/s00595-007-3541-5

[68] Orringer MB, Marshall B, Iannettoni MD. Eliminating the cervical esophagogastric anastomotic leak with a side-to-side stapled anastomosis. The Journal of Thoracic and Cardiovascular Surgery. 2000;**119**(2):277-288. DOI: 10.1016/S0022-5223(00)70183-8

[69] Turkyilmaz A, Eroglu A, Aydin Y, Tekinbas C, Muharrem Erol M, Karaoglanoglu N. The management of esophagogastric anastomotic leak after esophagectomy for esophagealcarcinoma. Diseases of the Esophagus. 2009;**22**(2):119-126. DOI: 10.1111/j.1442-2050.2008.00866.x

[70] Dai JG, Zhang ZY, Min JX, Huang XB, Wang JS. Wrapping of the omental pedicle flap around esophagogastric anastomosis after esophagectomy for esophageal cancer. Surgery (USA). 2011;**149**(3):404-410. DOI: 10.1016/j.surg.2010.08.005

[71] Bhat MA, Dar MA, Lone GN, Dar AM. Use of pedicledomentum in esophagogastric anastomosis for prevention of anastomotic leak. The Annals of Thoracic Surgery. 2006;**82**(5):1857-1862. DOI: 10.1016/j.athoracsur.2006.05.101

[72] Deitmar S, Anthoni C, Palmes D, Haier J, Senninger N, Brüwer M. Are leukocytes and CRP early indicators for anastomotic leakage after esophageal resection? Zentralblatt für Chirurgie. 2009;**134**(1):83-89. DOI: 10.1055/s-0028-1098768

[73] Veeramootoo D, Parameswaran R, Krishnadas R, et al. Classification and early recognition of gastric conduit failure after minimally invasive esophagectomy. Surgical Endoscopy. 2009;**23**(9):2110-2116. DOI: 10.1007/s00464-008-0233-1

[74] Sauvanet A, Baltar J, Le Mee J, Belghiti J. Diagnosis and conservative management of intrathoracic leakage after oesophagectomy. The British Journal of Surgery. 1998;**85**(10):1446-1449. DOI: 10.1046/j.1365-2168.1998.00869.x

[75] Roh S, Iannettoni MD, Keech JC, Bashir M, Gruber PJ, Parekh KR. Role of barium swallow in diagnosing clinically significant anastomotic leak following esophagectomy. Korean Journal of Thoracic and Cardiovascular Surgery. 2016;**49**(2):99-106. DOI: 10.5090/kjtcs.2016.49.2.99

[76] Andreou A, Struecker B, Biebl M, Pratschke J. Routine barium swallow may be unnecessary after resection of esophageal cancer. Journal of the American College of Surgeons. 2015;**221**(4):S145. DOI: 10.1016/j.jamcollsurg.2015.07.347

[77] Kauer WKH, Stein HJ, Dittler H, Siewert JR. Stent implantation as a treatment option in patients with thoracic anastomotic leaks after esophagectomy. Surgical Endoscopy. 2008;**22**(1):50-53. DOI: 10.1007/s00464-007-9504-5

[78] Brangewitz M, Voigtländer T, Helfritz FA, et al. Endoscopic closure of esophageal intrathoracic leaks: Stent versus endoscopic vacuum-assisted closure, a retrospective analysis. Endoscopy. 2013;**45**(6):433-438. DOI: 10.1055/s-0032-1326435

[79] Ahrens M, Schulte T, Egberts J, et al. Drainage of esophageal leakage using endoscopic vacuum therapy: A prospective pilot study. Endoscopy. 2010;**42**(9):693-698. DOI: 10.1055/s-0030-1255688

[80] Wedemeyer J, Brangewitz M, Kubicka S, et al. Management of major postsurgical gastroesophageal intrathoracic leaks with an endoscopic vacuum-assisted closure system. Gastrointestinal Endoscopy. 2010;**71**(2):382-386. DOI: 10.1016/j.gie.2009.07.011

[81] Mennigen R, Harting C, Lindner K, et al. Comparison of endoscopic vacuum therapy versus stent for anastomotic leak after esophagectomy. Journal of Gastrointestinal Surgery. 2015;**19**(7):1229-1235. DOI: 10.1007/s11605-015-2847-7

[82] Diddee R, Shaw IH. Acquired tracheo-oesophageal fistula in adults. Continuing Education in Anaesthesia Critical Care & Pain. 2006;**6**(3):105-108. DOI: 10.1093/bjaceaccp/mkl019

[83] Blackmon SH, Santora R, Schwarz P, Barroso A, Dunkin BJ. Utility of removable esophageal covered self-expanding metal stents for leak and fistula management. The Annals of Thoracic Surgery. 2010;**89**(3):931-937. DOI: 10.1016/j.athoracsur.2009.10.061

[84] Marchese S, Qureshi YA, Hafiz SP, et al. Intraoperative pyloric interventions during oesophagectomy: A multicentre study. Journal of Gastrointestinal Surgery. 2018:1-6. DOI: 10.1007/s11605-018-3759-0

[85] Eldaif SM, Lee R, Adams KN, et al. Intrapyloric botulinum injection increases postoperative esophagectomy complications. The Annals of Thoracic Surgery. 2014;**97**(6):1959-1965. DOI: 10.1016/j.athoracsur.2013.11.026

[86] Zhang L, Hou S, Miao J, Lee H. Risk factors for delayed gastric emptying in patients undergoing esophagectomy without pyloric drainage. The Journal of Surgical Research. 2017;**213**:46-50. DOI: 10.1016/j.jss.2017.02.012

[87] Smoke A, Delegge MH. Chyle leaks: Consensus on management? Nutrition in Clinical Practice. 2008;**23**(5):529-532. DOI: 10.1177/0884533608323424

[88] Jensen GL, Mascioli EA, Meyer LP, et al. Dietary modification of chyle composition in chylothorax. Gastroenterology. 1989;**97**(3):761-765. DOI: 10.1016/0016-5085(89)90650-1

[89] Dugue L, Sauvanet A, Farges O, Goharin A, Le Mee J, Belghiti J. Output of chyle as an indicator of treatment for chylothorax complicating oesophagectomy. The British Journal of Surgery. 1998;**85**(8):1147-1149. DOI: 10.1046/j.1365-2168.1998.00819.x

[90] Lin Y, Li Z, Li G, et al. Selective en masse ligation of the thoracic duct to prevent chyle leak after esophagectomy. The Annals of Thoracic Surgery. 2017;**103**(6):1802-1807

[91] Shackcloth MJ, Poullis M, Lu J, Page RD. Preventing of chylothorax after oesophagectomy by routine pre-operative administration of oral cream. European Journal of Cardio-Thoracic Surgery. 2001;**20**(5):1035-1036. DOI: 10.1016/S1010-7940(01)00928-9

[92] Sriram K, Meguid RA, Meguid MM. Nutritional support in adults with chyle leaks. Nutrition. 2016;**32**(2):281-286. DOI: 10.1016/j.nut.2015.08.002

[93] Browse NL, Allen DR, Wilson NM. Management of chylothorax. The British Journal of Surgery. 1997;**84**(12):1711-1716. DOI: 10.1046/j.1365-2168.1997.02858.x

[94] Martucci N, Tracey M, Rocco G. Postoperative chylothorax. Thoracic Surgery Clinics. Nov. 2015;**25**(4):523-528

[95] Zabeck H, Muley TF, Dienemann HF, Hoffmann H. Management of chylothorax in adults: When is surgery indicated? The Thoracic and Cardiovascular Surgeon. 2011; **59**(4): 243-246

[96] Nair SK, Petko M, Hayward MP. Aetiology and management of chylothorax in adults. European Journal of Cardio-Thoracic Surgery. 2007;**32**(2):362-369. DOI: 10.1016/j.ejcts.2007.04.024

[97] Pamarthi V, Stecker MS, Schenker MP, et al. Thoracic duct embolization and disruption for treatment of chylous effusions: Experience with 105 patients. Journal of Vascular and Interventional Radiology. 2014;**25**(9):1398-1404. DOI: 10.1016/j.jvir.2014.03.027

[98] Guevara CJ, Rialon KL, Ramaswamy RS, Kim SK, Darcy MD. US-guided, direct puncture retrograde thoracic duct access, lymphangiography, and embolization: Feasibility and efficacy. Journal of Vascular and Interventional Radiology. Dec. 2016;**27**(12):1890-1896

Chapter 4

The Clinical Relevance of Gastroesophageal Reflux Disease and Laryngopharyngeal Reflux in Clinical Practice

Aragona Salvatore Emanuele,
Mereghetti Giada and Giorgio Ciprandi

Additional information is available at the end of the chapter

http://dx.doi.org/10.5772/intechopen.78357

Abstract

Gastric reflux may be considered a para-physiological event that may occur up to 50 times a day. It usually happens when gas (less commonly liquids) flow back from stomach into esophagus. However, when defense mechanisms leave, disease may progress. If the esophagus is the trigger, gastroesophageal reflux disease (GERD) emerges. The prevalence of GERD in the primary care setting seems to be even more evident when one considers that, in the United States, 4.6 million office encounters annually are primarily for GERD, whereas 9.1 million encounters include GERD in the top 3 diagnoses for the encounter. GERD constitutes also the most frequently first-listed gastrointestinal diagnosis in ambulatory care visits. In addition, the extraesophageal manifestations of reflux, including LPR, asthma, and chronic cough, have been estimated to cost $5438 per patient in direct medical expenses in the first year after presentation and $13,700 for 5 years. Presently, the newest alginate compounds renowned the interest in this attracting and stimulating area. In this regard, a new medical device (Marial®), unique still now possessing the indication for both GERD and LPR, has been recently launched in the Italian market, two large surveys were conducted in Italy: RELIEF, involving 86 otolaryngologists, and EMERGE, involving 56 gastroenterologists. The aims of these surveys were: (1) to define clinical characteristics, including previous treatment, of the patients referred to consultation; (2) to evaluate the reliability of RFS, GIS, and RSI questionnaires in real-world settings, such as specialist office; and (3) to investigate the patients' perception of efficacy of the prescribed therapy, based on the best practice and considering also the new medical device Comparing the patients' perception of treatment efficacy, reduction in RSI values for each single symptom before and after a 4 week-treatment with Marial® alone or with PPI in add-on in EMERGE and RELIEF patients are reported. Marial® alone treatment induced a statistically significant higher reduction in each single symptom in RELIEF patients than in EMERGE patients, with the exception of heartburn, chest pain, indigestion, or stomach

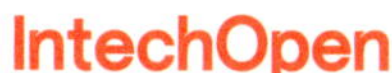

acid coming up. Similar results were obtained evaluating the reduction in RSI values in patients treated with PPI in add-on that was able to determine a higher statistically significant decrease in RELIEF than in EMERGE patients in each single symptom, with the exception of heartburn, chest pain, indigestion, or stomach acid coming up.

Keywords: regenerative medicine, GERD, LPR

1. Background

Actually, gastric reflux may be considered a para-physiological event that may occur up to 50 times a day. It usually happens when gas (less commonly liquids) flow back from stomach into esophagus. However, when defense mechanisms leave, disease may progress. If the esophagus is the trigger, gastroesophageal reflux disease (GERD) emerges. On the other hand, laryngopharyngeal reflux (LPR) is considered an extraesophageal manifestation of the GERD. Both GERD and its extraesophageal manifestation are very common in clinical practice. Both disorders have a relevant burden for the society: many pharmaco-economic studies were conducted in the United States. In population-based studies, 19.8% of North Americans complain of GERD symptoms, including heartburn and regurgitation, at least weekly [1]. Likewise, in the late 1990s, GERD accounted for $9.3 to $12.1 billion in direct annual healthcare costs in the United States, higher than any other digestive disease. Consequently, acid-suppressive agents are still the leading pharmaceutical expenditure in the United States.

The prevalence of GERD in the primary care setting seems to be even more evident when one considers that, in the United States, 4.6 million office encounters annually are primarily for GERD, whereas 9.1 million encounters include GERD in the top 3 diagnoses for the encounter. GERD constitutes also the most frequently first-listed gastrointestinal diagnosis in ambulatory care visits [2, 3]. In addition, the extraesophageal manifestations of reflux, including LPR, asthma, and chronic cough, have been estimated to cost $5438 per patient in direct medical expenses in the first year after presentation and $13,700 for 5 years. Estimates of the economic burden of extraesophageal reflux have shown that expenditures for extraesophageal manifestations of reflux could surpass $50 billion, 86% of which could be attributable to pharmaceutical costs [2, 3]. In addition, the National Health Care Survey carried out by the Center for Disease Control and Prevention has reported that the main complaint for primary care patient visits was cough in 6.1%, throat symptoms in 4%, and asthma in 2.8% [4]. Within these visits for cough, asthma, and throat symptoms are contained the hidden prevalence of extraesophageal manifestations of GERD, which to date have not been adequately addressed from a medical or surgical perspective due to their perceived obscurity. Therefore, the gastric reflux, globally understood, represents a very important medical issue that deserves adequate attention in daily practice.

From a pathophysiological point of view, gastric reflux includes different mechanisms, such as the provocation and perception of reflux. The transient lower esophageal sphincter relaxations (TLESR), hiatus hernia, acid pocket, visceral hypersensitivity, and obesity represent important causes of gastric reflux. Impaired esophageal, and extraesophageal, mucosal integrity, poor esophageal clearance, and delayed gastric emptying could be associated with GERD development. In addition, another pathogenic factor is a neural reflex sustained by acid exposure: the so-called Reflex-Reflux [5].

Distinguishing whether cough, LPR, and asthma may be sustained by GERD remains difficult challenging for both the primary care physician and the specialist. The distinction between them is clinically relevant as treatment of GERD with the intent of improving or curing extraesophageal manifestation could be ineffective. To review the current literature on extraesophageal manifestations of reflux should assist in clinical decision making.

The Montreal Classification gave the most recent consensus definition of GERD. This document defines GERD as heartburn symptoms or complications resulting from the reflux of gastric contents into the esophagus, up to the oral cavity, and lungs [5]. GERD is again classified into two subgroups. The first subgroup is represented by GERD with heartburn symptoms but without endoscopic evidence of mucosal erosions (the so called Non-Erosive Reflux Disease or NERD). The second sub-group is GERD with heartburn symptoms accompanied by objective evidence of erosions, ulcers, and inflammation (the so called Erosive Reflux Disease or ERD) [6].

It has to be considered that functional heartburn might fall under endoscopic negative disease. However, it is important to note that it is a distinct entity from NERD. NERD is usually defined as typical reflux symptoms without evidence of reflux disease in endoscopy but abnormal acid exposure on the impedance-pH monitoring and is responsive to proton pump inhibitors - PPI [7, 8]. Functional heartburn on the other hand, as defined by Rome IV classification, is a retrosternal burning discomfort or pain refractory to anti-secretory therapy without presence of GERD, histopathologic abnormality, motility disorder or structural abnormality for at least 3 months with symptoms onset at least 6 months prior to the diagnosis [5].

As just defined, stomach content may also reflux outside of the esophagus into respiratory organs, such as extraesophageal reflux, including LPR. LPR is most commonly manifested as laryngeal symptoms such as coughing, hoarseness, dysphagia, globus, and sore throat, but there can be signs also of nose, sinus, ear, and eye involvement [9]. Epidemiological studies have shown that the prevalence of this LPR may be extremely high, that it has certain characteristics of an outbreak and that it is one of the most common causes of patient visits to their family medicine physicians, but also to otolaryngologists, gastroenterologists, pediatricians, pulmonologists, allergists, and psychiatrists [1, 10–13]. Today it has been proven that gastroesophageal reflux is not the only cause of LPR. LPR is a multifactorial syndrome with a vast clinical representation, during the disease and with complications, so it requires and deserves a multidisciplinary approach. Based on newly discovered findings about the specific pathogenesis of the disease, LPR may be considered a new clinical entity [11–13]. As once pointed out, GERD is caused by the lower esophageal sphincter dysfunction and the dysfunction of the stomach emptying mechanism. Esophageal mucosa has protective mechanisms against aggressive factors of the stomach content (mucosal barrier) and it remains intact when a physiological reflux occurs, which normally happens at night. However, laryngeal and pharyngeal mucosa do not possess the esophageal protective mechanisms, so acid and peptic activity of the stomach content quickly leads to mucosal lesions. Notably, laryngopharyngeal reflux occurs most commonly during the day as a result of the upper esophageal sphincter dysfunction. This aspect is intriguing as typical GERD symptoms usually occur in supine position and overnight. However, acidity of the stomach content is not the only cause of LPR. Pepsin with its proteolytic effects can be the determining factor. Other possible etiological factors are pancreatic proteolytic enzymes, bile salts, and bacteria [1, 13, 14]. Extraesophageal manifestations of stomach content reflux have only recently started being seen as important based on the assumption of their important role in causing respiratory tract diseases. In clinical practice, LPR is mostly not recognized because it may be a "silent reflux" and diagnostic and therapeutic protocols are still inadequate, so proper treatment is usually delayed. Laryngeal symptoms are the most common, so patients are managed by otolaryngologists. Indeed, otolaryngologists have developed the diagnostic Reflux Symptom Index (RSI) questionnaire based on the importance of certain disease symptoms and the Reflux Finding Score (RFS) based on frequency of pathological changes determined by laryngoscopy [15]. On the other hand, considering the high prevalence of the disease and uncharacteristic clinical image, most patients report to their family medicine physicians [14–17]. For family medicine physicians LPR represents an important medical problem and a challenge in fast diagnostics, proper treatment, and proper selection of patients who require additional multidisciplinary diagnostic procedures. Knowledge of pathogenic pathway of the disease and its clinical manifestations can help physicians in creating an adequate program for prevention, early diagnosis, and adequate therapy for LPR. In particular, it has to be considered that untreated LPR can be one of the etiological causes of laryngeal cancer. The development of the disease can be benign or malignant and life threatening, and all of its forms can considerably affect life quality in patients. Laryngeal pathological changes could be discovered with laryngoscopy, and some even with detailed esophagogastroscopy. These changes may include: edema, hyperemia, or erythema of the vocal chords and laryngeal edges, ventricular obliteration, granulation, presence of dense endolaryngeal secretion, and hypertrophy of the posterior commissure [10, 15]. As consequence, an appropriate diagnosis of LPR represents a challenge for general practitioner and specialists. A large number of clinical studies confirmed low specificity and sensitivity of diagnostic tests such as laryngoscopy, esophagogastroscopy, proximal pH monitoring (hypopharyngeal and oropharyngeal). Evaluation of symptoms using the Reflux Symptom Index is considered to be the basic diagnostic procedure. A newer method of measuring salivary pepsin (Pep-test) can confirm LPR diagnosis because its sensitivity and specificity is 87% [13]. In this regard, it has to be noted that pepsinogen is produced only in the stomach, so pepsin may be envisaged as a specific biomarker for gastric reflux. The Pep-test is a fast and non-invasive method and could have a wide variety of uses in primary health care.

LPR therapy is complex and requires also modification of the patient's lifestyle and habits. Body weight reduction and physical activity, quitting cigarettes and alcohol use are one of the first steps in lowering the intensity of symptoms in patients [17]. Nutritional interventions with correct food choices and bowel movement regulation lead to lowering dyspeptic complains, but also lower the number of reflux episodes. Emptying of the bowels causes lower intra-abdominal pressure, which leads to lower possibility of stomach content reflux into the esophagus, larynx and pharynx. Obesity, or more precisely high BMI, so including overweight, is an independent factor in stomach reflux occurrence because of its specific effect mechanism on the gastroesophageal juncture [17]. LPR treatment and management is supposed to reduce the acidity or stomach contents and neutralize acid-peptic activity in larynx, pharynx and esophagus. High dosages of PPI (proton pump inhibitors) have shown the best effects in reducing reflux in the course of 24 h. Alkaline water and alginates show a positive additional effect in lowering acid-peptic activity in the larynx and pharynx. Patients are supposed to have long-term treatment during the course of 6 months because of high sensitivity of the mucosal membrane in the stomach and pharynx. Difficult cases with a proven hiatal hernia can be considered for surgical treatment as well [6].

Therefore, acid suppression is the mainstay of therapy for gastric reflux, and PPIs are the most effective drug in this approach [18, 19]. Although PPIs are the treatment of choice for GERD, still approximately one-third of patients with GERD fail to respond symptomatically to a standard dose PPI, either partially or completely [20]. Actually, NERD accounts for 60–70% of GERD patients and is considered the most common presentation of GERD. However, only approximately 30–40% of NERD patients respond to a standard dose of PPIs, much lower than that in erosive esophagitis, and the low response rate to PPIs in NERD patients is the main contributor to the high portion of PPI failure phenomenon in GERD, and also LPR, management [21]. The mechanisms of failure of PPI therapy are complex and multifactorial [20, 22–24]. Consequently, other medications should be considered and used. In this context, alginates and histamine type-2 receptor antagonists (H2RAs) may provide additional benefit for symptom relief in patients with persistent symptoms despite PPI therapy and can be considered as add-on therapy for patients who fail with a PPI. However, because of the concern about tolerance, H2RA is suggested to be taken on demand or intermittently. PPI-refractory GERD (and LPR), defined as persistent reflux symptoms not responding to a double dose of a PPI therapy during a treatment period of at least 12 weeks, is an important issue in clinical practice and poses a great challenge for general practitioners, internists, gastroenterologists, and otolaryngologists [20]. Compliance with therapy should be verified first by the physician, and the presence of functional gastrointestinal disorders, psychological distress, functional heartburn or other esophagitis not related to reflux should also be carefully evaluated in these patients.

On the basis of these concepts, alginate may be considered a fruitful and relevant option in many patients with reflux disease. In particular, the knowledge about the utility of alginates derives from an interesting research area investigating the pathogenic role of the so-called "acid pocket." The acid pocket is a short zone of unbuffered highly acidic gastric juice that accumulates in the proximal stomach after meals. Serving as the source of acid reflux, the acid pocket increases the propensity for acid reflux by all conventional mechanisms, such as TLESR and hiatus hernia, and has been considered as an important cause of GERD [25, 26]. Alginate is an anionic polysaccharide occurring naturally in brown algae and has a unique property in the treatment of gastric reflux by eliminating the acid pocket. Alginate-antacid formulation can reduce postprandial symptoms by neutralizing the acidity of gastric contents. In addition to neutralizing the gastric acidity, more importantly, alginate and bicarbonate, usually contained in an alginate-based formulation, form a foamy gel that is like a raft floating on the surface of gastric contents after interacting with gastric acid, and this barrier-like gel displaces the acid pocket from the esophageal-gastric junction and protects both the esophageal and the upper respiratory mucosa from the acid and non-acid reflux by gel coating [27–30]. Like an antacid, an alginate-based formulation demonstrates an immediate onset of effect within 1 h of administration, which is faster than a PPI and H2RA [31]. Compared with antacids, an alginate-based formulation is more effective than an antacid in controlling postprandial esophageal acid exposure and quickly relieving reflux symptoms, including heartburn, regurgitation, vomiting and belching, with longer duration [32–34]. Alginate-based formulations are also non-inferior to omeprazole in achieving a heartburn-free period in moderate episodic heartburn [35]. Therefore, alginate has the special properties of protection of the esophageal and upper respiratory mucosa from acid and non-acid reflux and displacement of acid pocket away from the esophagus, all of which make alginate an attractive agent in the management of refractory reflux symptoms with a cause other than by acid, such as NERD [36]. Compared with placebo, an alginate-antacid formulation demonstrated superior relief of reflux symptoms including heartburn and regurgitation in both patients with NERD and erosive esophagitis in a double-blind randomized controlled trial [37]. In another double-blind randomized clinical trial comparing the efficacy of alginate to omeprazole in patients with NERD, alginate demonstrated non-inferiority to omeprazole and was as effective as omeprazole for symptomatic relief [38]. Furthermore, adding alginate to a PPI can significantly relieve heartburn compared to using a PPI alone in patients with NERD, suggesting an additional benefit of alginate as add-on therapy in the management of refractory symptoms [39].

Interestingly, in a meta-analysis study, six of nine randomized trials found no difference between the PPI and placebo groups for LPR, whereas three trials exhibited statistically significant results [1]. In a systemic review, three of four randomized controlled studies revealed that prokinetic agents significantly reduced LPR symptoms, but there were too many study limitations to draw firm conclusions [40]. In a small randomized controlled study, a liquid alginate suspension could achieve significant improvement in the symptom scores and clinical findings of LPR [41].

Therefore, on the basis of this discussed background, the management of suspected LPR is intriguing as it is very difficult, if even possible, to make a definitive diagnosis with the tools currently available [42]. If there is no doubt that many patients do have LPR symptoms, the probability of suspecting LPR, especially when typical reflux symptoms are lacking and PPIs do not improve symptoms, are low, mainly in non-specialist setting. LPR management is responsible of high economic burden mainly related to the prescription of PPIs, which may be, in most cases, not justified [3, 43, 44]. Therefore, in patients, initially visited by GP, who do not respond to a 2 to 3-month course of double dose PPI therapy, the role of the otolaryngologist is to document the presence of signs and symptoms suggestive of LPR with appropriate (i.e., validated and reproducible) investigations, namely fiber-endoscopy, and validated questionnaire (for example RSI and RFS). If LPR is documented, it is reasonable empirically testing these patients on PPIs to check for reflux control may be useful to select PPI-responder patients. If PPI are not adequate to control symptoms an add-on treatment should be prescribed. On the basis of the above-mentioned concepts, alginate could be a first-choice option. As a matter of the fact, as there is no specific and focused medication able to irreversibly inactivate pepsin and block acid production, other compounds have place in LPR management, including medical devices with barrier effect. In the current scenario, an effective supportive strategy may be constituted by compounds able to strengthen the epithelial barrier providing protection from acid and pepsin and promoting mucosal healing. In other words, an old concept could be revised for LPR therapy: the "cytoprotection" of mucosal tissues [45]. Mucosal cytoprotection was an ideal target of two main drug classes: prostaglandins and sucralfate. Many clinical trials supported this theory that met favorable impression some decades ago [46–49].

Presently, the newest alginate compounds renowned the interest in this attracting and stimulating area. In this regard, a new medical device (Marial®), unique still now possessing the indication for both GERD and LPR, has been recently launched in the Italian market. It is an innovative gel compound, containing magnesium alginate and E-Gastryal® (hyaluronic acid, hydrolyzed keratin, Tara gum, and Xantana gum). E-Gastryal® is a complex of phyto-polymers, Tara and Xantana gums, that are natural polysaccharides with high molecular weight and partially hydrosoluble, and able to provide viscosity to the solution and to generate a support frame where keratin peptide chains and hyaluronic acid anchor. Hyaluronic acid (HA) is a biopolymer with medium molecular weight characterized by optimal hygroscopic and hydrodynamic features. The chemical–physical properties of the polymeric complex confer mucoadhesiveness to E-Gastryal® so increasing the contact surface and the residence time on the mucous membranes of larynx, pharynx, and esophagus. In this context, hyaluronic acid is extremely bioavailable and able to carries out its activity aimed to induce repairing and regenerating the damaged epithelium. HA, by its hydrophilic essence, realizes a favorable milieu for cellular migration; in addition, HA, having a scavenger activity of free radicals, exerts a protective role towards oxide damage and proteolytic enzymes, such as pepsin.

Hydrolyzed keratin, an indigestible substance, increases the solidity and the resistance of E-Gastryal®, enhancing the barrier effect. Really, keratin abounds with cysteine, amino acid sulfide, that forms disulfide bridges extremely firm and able to link the amino acid chains, making an helical structure characterized by difficult dissolution and resistant to attack of acid and pepsin. The alginate has the peculiar property of a boating raft at the acid pocket and selectively inhibits pepsin by mannuronic acid, highly contained in the specific alginate [50]. In particular, this medical device contains magnesium alginate with high ratio mannuronic acid/glucuronic acid and with raised viscosity shaping a stable and compact raft.

For these reasons, two large surveys were conducted in Italy, involving both otolaryngologists and gastroenterologists. The aims were to define the patients' characteristics, including the clinical features, the assessment of treatments, and new therapeutic approaches in view of the new medical device Marial®.

2. Clinical experience

As pointed out, the gastroesophageal reflux is considered a normal physiological process that usually happens after eating in healthy infants, children, young people and adults. In contrast, gastroesophageal reflux disease occurs when the effect of GER leads to symptoms severe enough to merit medical treatment. In clinical practice, it is difficult to differentiate between GER and GERD, and the terms are used interchangeably by health professionals and families alike. There is no simple, reliable and accurate diagnostic test to confirm whether the condition is GER or GERD, and this in turn affects research and clinical decisions [50–52]. Furthermore, the term GERD covers a number of specific conditions that have different effects and present in different ways. This makes it difficult to identify the person who genuinely has GERD, and to estimate the real prevalence and burden of the problem. Nevertheless, regardless of the definition used, GERD affects many subjects, who commonly seek advice from primary, secondary or tertiary care. As a result, it constitutes a major health burden for the Health Service. Moreover, if gastric refluxate moves more proximally into the laryngopharynx, it is defined laryngopharyngeal reflux (LPR). LPR should be considered as part of extraesophageal reflux (EER), reflux involving structures other than, or in addition to, the esophagus, and airway reflux involving proximal gastric reflux into the airways. LPR contributes to several otorhinolaryngologic symptoms and inflammatory disorders, and probably also to neoplastic diseases of the laryngopharynx, and seems to be also as common in children and infants as adults.

From a diagnostic point of view, GERD and LPR diagnosis may be performed on a clinical ground as there is no gold-standard diagnostic tool. In this regard, some questionnaires may very fruitful in clinical practice: Reflux Finding Score (RFS) based on signs viewed by laryngoscopy, Reflux Score Index (RSI) based on reflux symptoms, and GERD Impact Scale (GIS) based on frequency of symptoms, as reported in the tables (**Tables 1–3**).

	None of the time	**A little of the time**	**Some of the time**	**All of the time**
	1	**2**	**3**	**4**
In the past week				
1. How often have you had the following symptoms				
a. Pain in chest/behind the breastbone?				
b. Burning sensation in your chest or behind the breastbone?				
c. Regurgitation or acid taste in your mouth?				
d. Pain or burning in upper stomach?				
e. Sore throat or hoarseness that is related to your heartburn or acid reflux?				
2. How often have you had difficulty in getting a good night's sleep because of your symptoms?				
3. How often have your symptoms prevented you from eating or drinking any of the foods you like?				
4. How often have your symptoms kept you from being fully productive in your job or daily activities?				
5. How often do you take additional medication other than what the physician told you to take (such as Gaviscon, Maalox)?				

Table 1. GERD Impact Scale (GIS).

Within the last month, how did the following problems affect you?	**0 = no problem** **5 = severe problem**					
1. Hoarseness or a problem with your voice	0	1	2	3	4	5
2. Clearing your throat	0	1	2	3	4	5
3. Excess throat mucus or postnasal drip	0	1	2	3	4	5
4. Difficulty swallowing food, liquids, or pills	0	1	2	3	4	5
5. Coughing after you ate or after lying down	0	1	2	3	4	5
6. Breathing difficulties or choking episodes	0	1	2	3	4	5
7. Troublesome or annoying cough	0	1	2	3	4	5
8. Sensation of something sticking in your throat or a lump in your throat	0	1	2	3	4	5
9. Heartburn, chest pain, indigestion, or stomach acid coming up	0	1	2	3	4	5
RSI > 13 = Abnormal	Total					

Abbreviation: RSI, reflux symptom index.

Table 2. Reflux Symptom Index.

From a management point of view, the guidelines suggest to give advice about GER and reassure patients and caregivers. Patients with dyspepsia with mild–moderate symptoms and without severe complications, such as bleeding, painful complaints, vomiting, could be treated with empirical full-dose PPI therapy for 4 weeks. Patients with GERD could be treated with a full-dose PPI for 4 or 8 weeks. If symptoms recur after initial treatment, a PPI could be offered at the lowest dose possible to control symptoms. In addition, it is recommended to encourage people who need long-term management of dyspepsia symptoms to reduce their use of prescribed medication stepwise: by using the effective lowest dose, by trying 'as-needed' use when appropriate, and by returning to self-treatment with antacid and/or alginate therapy (unless there is an underlying condition or co-medication that needs continuing treatment). It is also necessary to advise people that it may be appropriate for them to return to self-treatment with antacid and/or alginate therapy (either prescribed or purchased over-the-counter and taken as needed). Finally, it is important to avoid long-term, frequent dose and continuous antacid therapy (it only relieves symptoms in the short term rather than preventing them).

On the basis of these considerations, proposed by guidelines, alginates may be considered as a valid and reasonable therapeutic option. A new medical device (Marial®), unique still now possessing the indication for both GERD and LPR, has been recently launched in the Italian market [53]. It is an innovative gel compound, containing magnesium alginate and E-Gastryal®. E-Gastryal® is a complex of phyto-polymers, keratin, Tara and Xantana gums, that are natural polysaccharides with high molecular weight and partially hydrosoluble, and able to provide viscosity to the solution and to generate a support frame where keratin peptide chains and hyaluronic acid anchor. Hyaluronic acid (HA) is a biopolymer with medium molecular weight characterized by optimal hygroscopic and hydrodynamic features. The chemical–physical properties of the polymeric complex confer mucoadhesiveness to E-Gastryal® so increasing the contact surface and the residence time on the mucous membranes of larynx, pharynx, and esophagus.

Subglottic edema	0 = absent
	2 = present
Ventricular edema	2 = partial
	4 = complete
Erythema/hyperemia	2 = arytenoids only
	4 = diffuse
Vocal-fold edema	1 = mild
	2 = moderate
	3 = severe
	4 = polypoid
Diffuse laryngeal edema	1 = mild
	2 = moderate
	3 = severe
	4 = obstructing
Posterior commissure hypertrophy	1 = mild
	2 = moderate
	3 = severe
	4 = obstructing
Granuloma/granulation tissue	0 = absent
	2 = present
Thicken laryngeal mucus	0 = absent
	2 = present

RFS, Reflux Finding Score. RFS > 7 suspect of laryngopharyngeal reflux (LPR).

Table 3. Reflux Finding Score.

Therefore, two large surveys were conducted in Italy: RELIEF, involving 86 otolaryngologists, and EMERGE, involving 56 gastroenterologists [54–56]. The aims of these surveys were: (1) to define clinical characteristics, including previous treatment, of the patients referred to consultation; (2) to evaluate the reliability of RFS, GIS, and RSI questionnaires in real-world settings, such as specialist office; and (3) to investigate the patients' perception of efficacy of the prescribed therapy, based on the best practice and considering also the new medical device.

The outcomes of these surveys are here presented and discussed. Now, we would draw the conclusive remarks from a pragmatic point of view. So, we compared the most relevant outcomes obtained by the two surveys.

First, we compared RSI questionnaires: at baseline, RSI questionnaire was filled by 1934 RELIEF patients and by 789 EMERGE patients. Globally, 594 (75.3%) EMERGE patients and 1250

(64.6%) RELIEF patients had positive RSI score. RSI values for each single symptom are analytically reported in **Figure 1**. The symptoms with the highest score were: heartburning, sensation of something sticking in the throat or a lump in the throat, and clearing throat, whereas breathing difficulties or choking episodes had the lowest score. The total score was 16 [14–20] in the EMERGE patients was significantly higher than in the RELIEFE patients: 16 [12–20] ($p < 0.001$; data not shown). Interestingly, RELIEF patients had significantly higher scores for some symptoms, including lump sensation, cough, dyspnea, hoarseness, and throat clearing, whereas EMERGE patients had higher scores for heartburn and difficult swallowing. So, the clinical features were really different in the two populations, such as GERD and LPR patients.

Considering the previous treatments, the frequency of past/current treatments in the EMERGE group (**Figure 2A**) was significantly higher than in RELIEF group (**Figure 2B**) patients ($p < 0.0001$): this outcome underlines the more intense recourse to medical therapy in GERD patients than in LPR patients. Analyzing the treatment options, **Figure 3** shows the distribution of different types of treatments prescribed in the past (panel A, C) or currently used (panel B, D): monotherapy with PPI, PPI in add-on, and Miscellany in EMERGE (panel A, B) and RELIEF (panel C, D) patients. LPR patients were more frequently treated with PPI as monotherapy and with miscellany treatments, whereas GERD patients use more commonly PPI plus add-on, even though PPI alone are the first-choice therapy also in GERD. Considering the distribution of the new prescribed

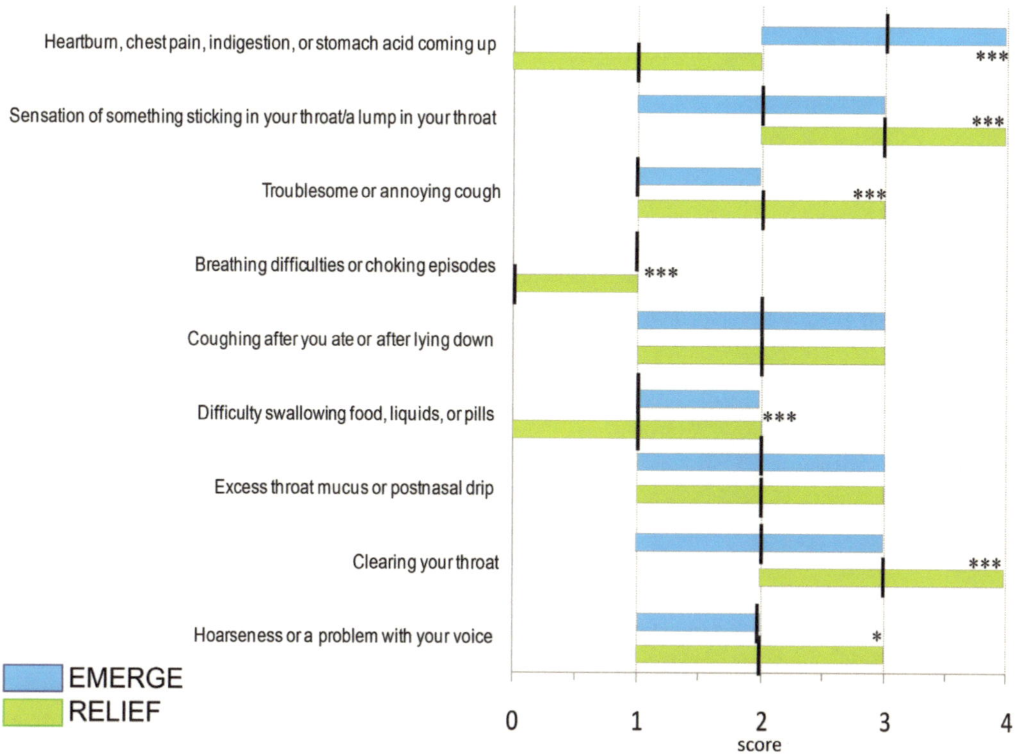

Figure 1. Reflux Symptom Index (RSI) as median values for each single symptom in the EMERGE (no. 789) and in the RELIEF population (no. 1934). Scores are reported as medians (bars) with lower and upper quartiles (boxes).

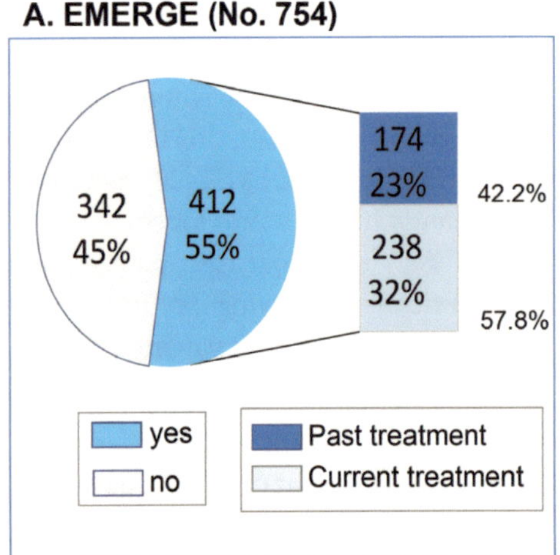

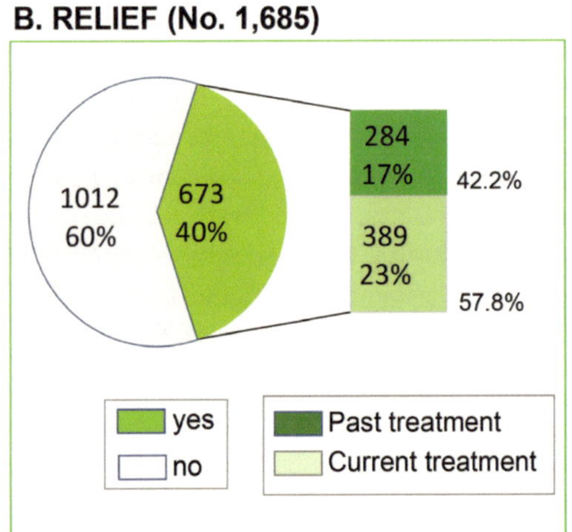

Figure 2. Distribution of the EMERGE (panel A) or RELIEF (panel B) patients according to the treatments: past, current, or never.

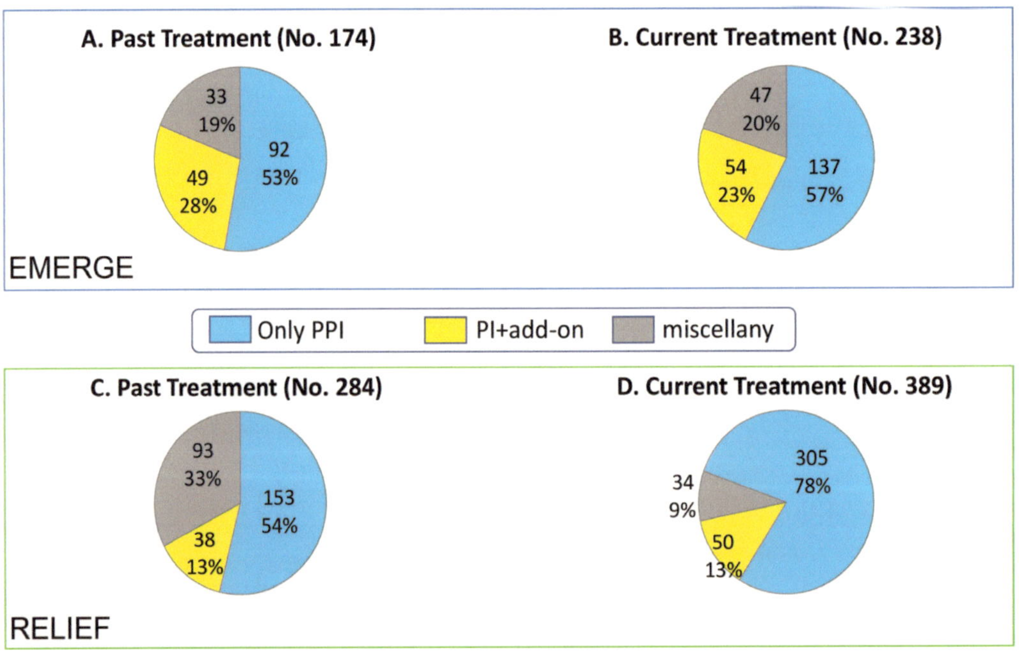

Figure 3. Distribution of different types of treatments prescribed in the past (panel A, C) or currently used (panel B, D): monotherapy with PPI, PPI in add-on, and miscellany in EMERGE (panel A, B) and RELIEF (panel C, D) patients.

treatments (i.e., prescriptions made during the visits) and specifically of Marial® as monotherapy, PPI as monotherapy or PPI in add-on, there was difference in EMERGE (**Figure 4A**) and in RELIEF (**Figure 4B**) patients ($p < 0.0001$): LPR patients were preferentially treated with Marial® alone, whereas GERD patients were treated essentially with PPI plus add-on.

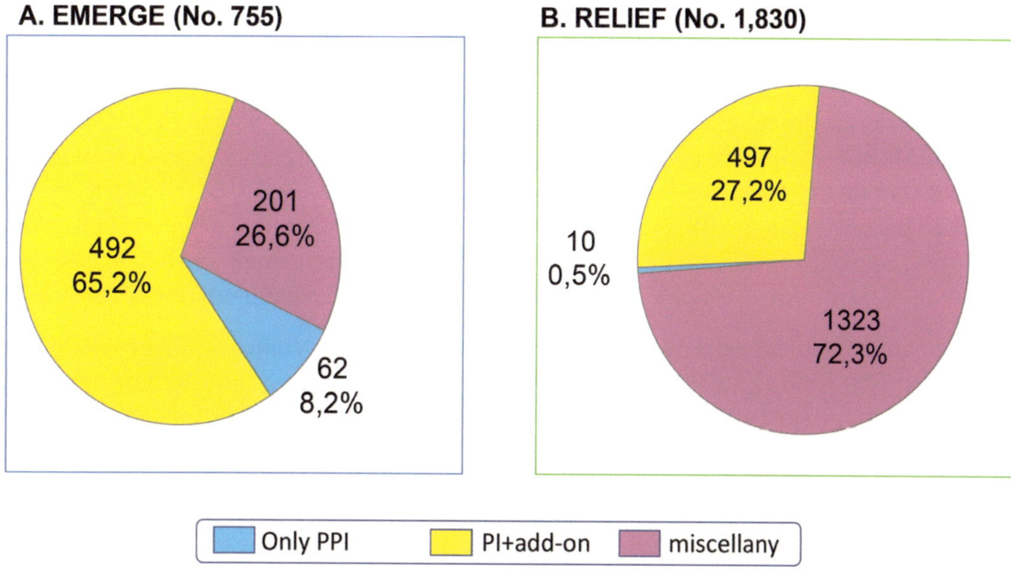

Figure 4. Distribution of the Marial® as monotherapy, PPI as monotherapy or PPI in add-on in new prescribed treatments (i.e., prescription during the visit) in EMERGE (panel A) and RELIEF (panel B) patients.

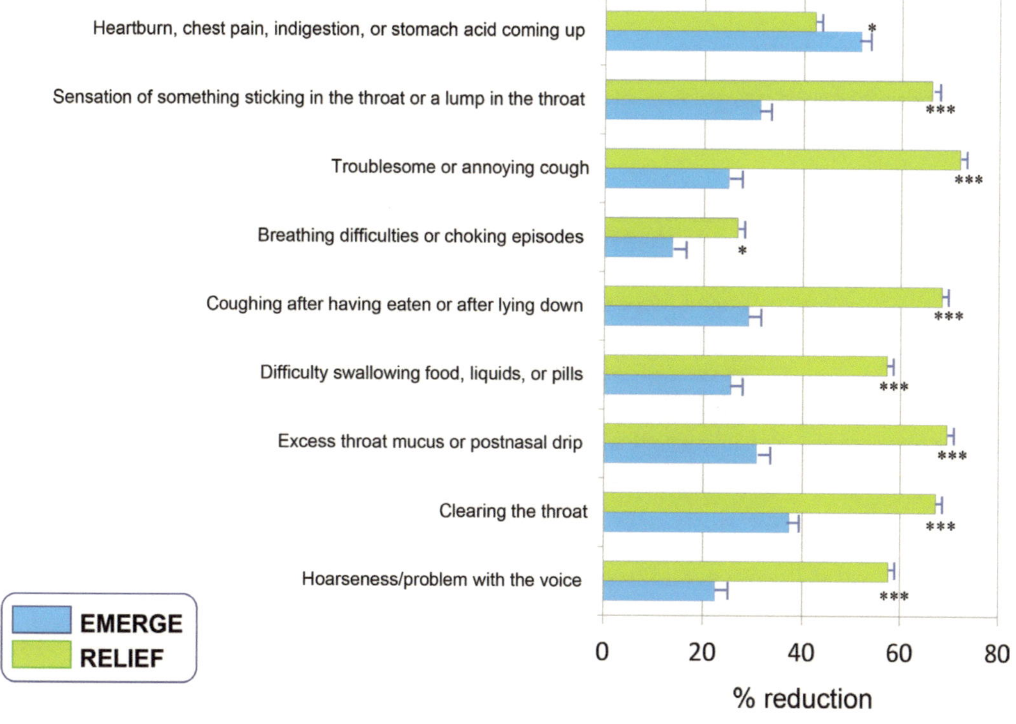

Figure 5. Reduction in RSI values for each single symptom before and after a 4 week-treatment with Marial® as monotherapy in EMERGE and in RELIEF patients.

Comparing the patients' perception of treatment efficacy, reduction in RSI values for each single symptom before and after a 4 week-treatment with Marial® alone or with PPI in add-on in EMERGE and RELIEF patients are reported in **Figures 5** and **6**. Marial® alone treatment induced a statistically significant higher reduction in each single symptom in RELIEF patients than in EMERGE patients, with the exception of heartburn, chest pain, indigestion, or stomach acid coming up (**Figure 5**). Similar results were obtained evaluating the reduction in RSI values in patients treated with PPI in add-on that was able to determine a higher statistically significant decrease in RELIEF than in EMERGE patients in each single symptom, with the exception of heartburn, chest pain, indigestion, or stomach acid coming up (**Figure 6**).

In conclusion, these two surveys provided some interesting outcomes: (i) diagnostic questionnaires (RSI, RFS, and GIS) are reliable and useful both during the visit and to orient the treatment decision; (ii) GERD and LPR present different clinical features; (iii) as consequence the treatments (both previous and actual) are different; (iv) the introduction of Marial® significantly affected the otolaryngologist approach and partially the gastroenterologist orientation; (v) Marial® was effective both in LPR and GERD patients; (vi) Marial® showed more effectiveness than conventional therapy (PPI plus add-on); and (vii) LPR patients were more responsive to medical treatments than GERD patients. Therefore, these outcomes may give a pragmatic usefulness to both otolaryngologists and gastroenterologists in clinical practice.

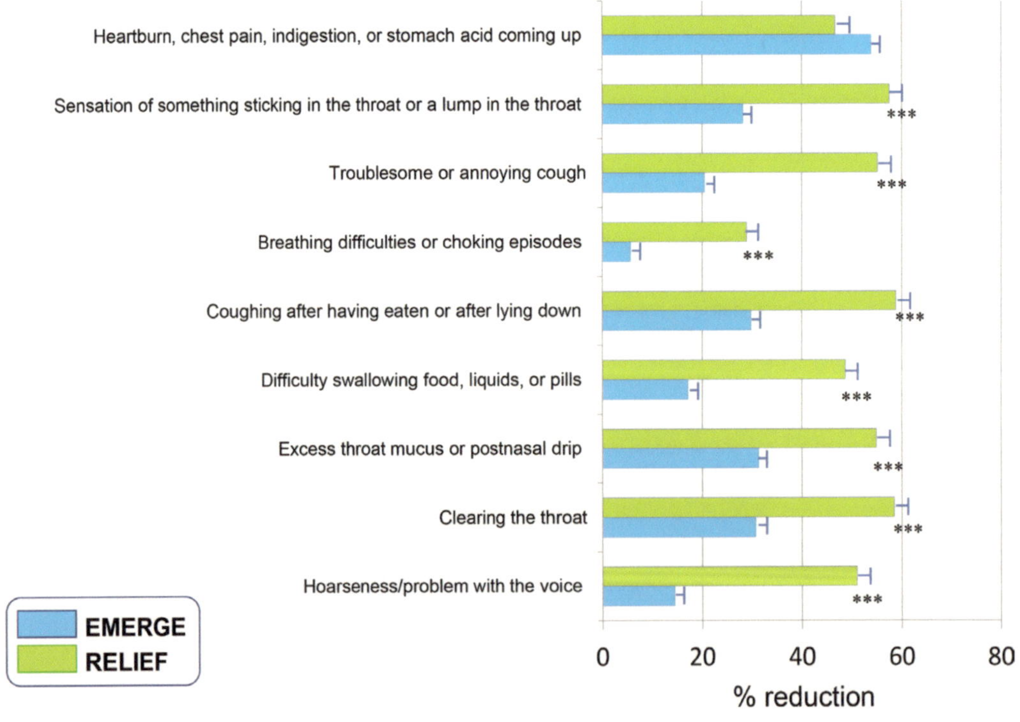

Figure 6. Reduction in RSI values for each single symptom before and after a 4 week-treatment with PPI + add-on in EMERGE and in RELIEF patients.

Author details

Aragona Salvatore Emanuele[1], Mereghetti Giada[1] and Giorgio Ciprandi[2]*

*Address all correspondence to: gio.cip@libero.it

1 Center of Regenerative Medicine, Humanitas Mater Domini, Castellanza (VA), Italy

2 Ospedale Policlinico San Martino, Genoa, Italy

References

[1] Sidhwa F, Moore A, Alligood E, Fisichella PM. Diagnosis and treatment of the extra-esophageal manifestations of gastroesophageal reflux disease. Annals of Surgery. 2017; **265**:63-67

[2] Rubenstein JH, Chen JW. Epidemiology of gastroesophageal reflux disease. Gastroenterology Clinics of North America. 2014;**43**:1-14

[3] Francis DO, Rymer JA, Slaughter JC, et al. High economic burden of caring for patients with suspected extraesophageal reflux. The American Journal of Gastroenterology. 2013;**108**:905-911

[4] Schappert SM, Burt CW. Ambulatory care visits to physician offices, hospital outpatient departments, and emergency departments: United States, 2001-02. Vital and Health Statistics. 2006:1-66

[5] Vakil N, van Zanten SV, Kahrilas P, Dent J, Jones R, Global Consensus Group. The Montreal definition and classification of gastroesophageal reflux disease: A global evidence-based consensus. The American Journal of Gastroenterology. 2006;**101**:1900-1920

[6] Katz P, Gerson LB. Corrigendum: Guidelines for the diagnosis and management of the gastroesophageal reflux disease. The American Journal of Gastroenterology. 2013;**108**: 308-328

[7] Savarino E. NERD: An umbrella term including heterogenous subpopulations. Nature Reviews. Gastroenterology & Hepatology. 2013;**10**:371-380

[8] Quasim A. Section II FGIDs: Diagnostic groups. Esophageal disorders. Gastroenterology. 2016;**150**:1368-1379

[9] Salihefendic N, Zidzic M, Cabric E. Laryngopharyngeal reflux disease—LPRD. Medical Archives. 2017;**71**:215-218

[10] Capagnolo AM, Priston J, Heidrichthoen R, Medeiros T, Assuncao RA. Laryngopharyngeal reflux: Diagnosis, treatment and latest research. International Archives of Otorhinolaryngology. 2014;**18**:184-191

[11] Dent J, El-Serag HB, Wallander MA, Johansson S. Epidemiology of gastroesophageal reflux disease: A systematic review. Gut. 2005;**54**:710-717

[12] Koufman JA. Laryngopharyngeal reflux 2002: A new paradigm of airway disease. Ear, Nose, & Throat Journal 2004; (Suppl. 1):10-29

[13] Saritas Yuksel E, Vaezi MF. New developments in extraesophageal reflux disease. Gastroenterología y Hepatología. 2012;**8**:590-599

[14] Barry DW, Vaezi MF. Laryngopharyngeal reflux: More questions than answers. Cleveland Clinic Journal of Medicine. 2010;**77**:327-334

[15] Belafsky PC, Postma GN, Amin MR, Koufman JA. Symptoms and findings of laryngopharyngeal reflux. Ear, Nose, & Throat Journal 2004; (Suppl. 1):30-39

[16] Abou-Ismail A, Vaezi MF. Evaluation of patients withsuspected laryngopharyngeal reflux: A practical approach. Current Gastroenterology Reports. 2011;**13**:213-218

[17] Martinucci I, de Bortoli N, Savarino E, Nacci A, Romeo SO, Bellini M, Savarino V, Fattori B, Marchi S. Optimal treatment of laryngopharyngeal reflux disease. Therapeutic Advances in Chronic Disease. 2013;**4**:287-301

[18] Kung YM, Hsu WH, Wu MC, Wang JW, Liu CJ, Su YC, et al. Recent advances in the pharmacological management of gastroesophageal reflux disease. Digestive Diseases and Sciences. 2017;**62**:3298-3316

[19] Sigterman KE, van Pinxteren B, Bonis PA, Lau J, Numans ME. Short-term treatment with proton pump inhibitors, H2-receptor antagonists and prokinetics for gastroesophageal reflux disease-like symptoms and endoscopy negative reflux disease. Cochrane Database of Systematic Reviews. 2013:CD002095

[20] Sifrim D, Zerbib F. Diagnosis and management of patients with reflux symptoms refractory to proton pump inhibitors. Gut. 2012;**61**:1340-1354

[21] Fass R, Shapiro M, Dekel R, Sewell J. Systematic review: Proton-pump inhibitor failure in gastro-oesophageal reflux disease—Where next? Alimentary Pharmacology & Therapeutics. 2005;**22**:79-94

[22] Fass R. Proton-pump inhibitor therapy in patients with gastrooesophageal reflux disease: Putative mechanisms of failure. Drugs. 2007;**67**:1521-1530

[23] Fass R, Gasiorowska A. Refractory GERD: What is it? Current Gastroenterology Reports. 2008;**10**:252-257

[24] Scarpellini E, Ang D, Pauwels A, et al. Management of refractory typical GERD symptoms. Nature Reviews. Gastroenterology & Hepatology. 2016;**13**:281-294

[25] Kahrilas PJ, McColl K, Fox M, et al. The acid pocket: A target for treatment in reflux disease? The American Journal of Gastroenterology. 2013;**108**:1058-1064

[26] Mitchell DR, Derakhshan MH, Robertson EV, McColl KE. The role of the acid pocket in gastroesophageal reflux disease. Journal of Clinical Gastroenterology. 2016;**50**:111-119

[27] Strugala V, Avis J, Jolliffe IG, Johnstone LM, Dettmar PW. The role of an alginate suspension on pepsin and bile acids–key aggressors in the gastric refluxate. Does this have implications for the treatment of gastro-oesophageal reflux disease? The Journal of Pharmacy and Pharmacology. 2009;**61**:1021-1028

[28] Kwiatek MA, Roman S, Fareeduddin A, Pandolfino JE, Kahrilas PJ. An alginate-antacid formulation (Gaviscon double action liquid) can eliminate or displace the postprandial 'acid pocket' in symptomatic GERD patients. Alimentary Pharmacology & Therapeutics. 2011;**34**:59-66

[29] Rohof WO, Bennink RJ, Smout AJ, Thomas E, Boeckxstaens GE. An alginate-antacid formulation localizes to the acid pocket to reduce acid reflux in patients with gastroesophageal reflux disease. Clinical Gastroenterology and Hepatology. 2013;**11**:1585-1591

[30] Sweis R, Kaufman E, Anggiansah A, et al. Post-prandial reflux suppression by a raft-forming alginate (Gaviscon advance) compared to a simple antacid documented by magnetic resonance imaging and pH-impedance monitoring: Mechanistic assessment in healthy volunteers and randomised, controlled, double-blind study in reflux patients. Alimentary Pharmacology & Therapeutics. 2013;**37**:1093-1102

[31] Dettmar PW, Sykes J, Little SL, Bryan J. Rapid onset of effect of sodium alginate on gastro-oesophageal reflux compared with ranitidine and omeprazole, and relationship between symptoms and reflux episodes. International Journal of Clinical Practice. 2006;**60**:275-283

[32] De Ruigh A, Roman S, Chen J, Pandolfino JE, Kahrilas PJ. Gaviscon double action liquid (antacid & alginate) is more effective than antacid in controlling post-prandial oesophageal acid exposure in GERD patients: A double-blind crossover study. Alimentary Pharmacology & Therapeutics. 2014;**40**:531-537

[33] Mandel KG, Daggy BP, Brodie DA, Jacoby HI. Review article: Alginate-raft formulations in the treatment of heartburn and acid reflux. Alimentary Pharmacology & Therapeutics. 2000;**14**:669-690

[34] Lai IR, Wu MS, Lin JT. Prospective, randomized, and active controlled study of the efficacy of alginic acid and antacid in the treatment of patients with endoscopy-negative reflux disease. World Journal of Gastroenterology. 2006;**12**:747-754

[35] Pouchain D, Bigard MA, Liard F, et al. Gaviscon(R) vs. omeprazole in symptomatic treatment of moderate gastroesophageal reflux. A direct comparative randomised trial. BMC Gastroenterology. 2012;**12**:18

[36] Woodland P, Lee C, Duraisamy Y, et al. Assessment and protection of esophageal mucosal integrity in patients with heartburn without esophagitis. The American Journal of Gastroenterology. 2013;**108**:535-543

[37] Sun J, Yang C, Zhao H, et al. Randomised clinical trial: The clinical efficacy and safety of an alginate-antacid (Gaviscon double action) versus placebo, for decreasing upper gastrointestinal symptoms in symptomatic gastroesophageal reflux disease (GERD) in China. Alimentary Pharmacology & Therapeutics. 2015;**42**:845-854

[38] Chiu CT, Hsu CM, Wang CC, et al. Randomised clinical trial: Sodium alginate oral suspension is non-inferior to omeprazole in the treatment of patients with non-erosive gastroesophageal disease. Alimentary Pharmacology & Therapeutics. 2013;**38**:1054-1064

[39] Manabe N, Haruma K, Ito M, et al. Efficacy of adding sodium alginate to omeprazole in patients with nonerosive reflux disease: A randomized clinical trial. Diseases of the Esophagus. 2012;**25**:373-380

[40] Glicksman JT, Mick PT, Fung K, Carroll TL. Prokinetic agents and laryngopharyngeal reflux disease: A systematic review. Laryngoscope. 2014;**124**:2375-2379

[41] McGlashan JA, Johnstone LM, Sykes J, Strugala V, Dettmar PW. The value of a liquid alginate suspension (Gaviscon advance) in the management of laryngopharyngeal reflux. European Archives of Oto-Rhino-Laryngology. 2009;**266**:243-251

[42] Zerbib F, Dulery C. Facts and fantasies on extraesophageal reflux. A gastroenterologist perspective. Journal of Clinical Gastroenterology. 2017;**51**:769-776

[43] Vertigan AE, Bone SL, Gibson PG. Laryngeal sensory dysfunction in laryngeal hypersensitivity syndrome. Respirology. 2013;**18**:948-956

[44] Aziz Q, Fass R, Gyawali CP. Functional esophageal disorders. Gastroenterology. In press. DOI: 10.1053/j.gastro.2016.02.012. [Epub ahead of print]

[45] Miller TA, Jacobson ED. Gastrointestinal cytoprotection by prostaglandins. Gut. 1979; **20**:75-87

[46] Johansson C, Bergström S. Prostaglandin and protection of the gastroduodenal mucosa. Scandinavian Journal of Gastroenterology. 1982;**77**:21-46

[47] Tasman-Jones C. Pathogenesis of peptic ulcer disease and gastritis: Importance of aggressive and cytoprotective factors. Scandinavian Journal of Gastroenterology. 1986: **122**:1-122:5

[48] Orlando RC. Cytoprotection by sucralfate in acid-exposed esophagus: A review. Scandinavian Journal of Gastroenterology. 1987;**127**:97-100

[49] Lauritsen K, Rask-Madsen J. Peptic ulcer disease, cytoprotection, and prostaglandins. Archives of Internal Medicine. 1990;**150**:695-701

[50] Chater PI, Wilcox MD, Brownlee IA. Alginate as a protease inhibitor in vitro and in a model gut system: Selective inhibition of pepsin but not trypsin. Carbohydrate Polymers. 2015;**131**:142-151

[51] Internal Clinical Guidelines Team (UK). Dyspepsia and Gastro-Oesophageal Reflux Disease: Investigation and Management of Dyspepsia, Symptoms Suggestive of Gastro-Oesophageal Reflux Disease, or Both. London: National Institute for Health and Care Excellence (UK); 2014 Sep

[52] Davies I, Burman-Roy S, Murphy MS, Guideline Development Group. Gastro-oesophageal reflux disease in children: NICE guidance. BMJ. 2015;**350**:7703

[53] Aragona SE, Mereghetti G, Ciprandi G. The gastric reflux: the therapeutical role of Marial. Journal of Biological Regulators and Homeostatic Agents. 2018 Apr 26;**32**(4). [Epub ahead of print]

[54] Bianchetti M, Peralta S, Nicita R, Aragona SE, Ciprandi G. The EMERGE (emerging from Gastroesophageal Reflux): an Italian survey—I. The viewpoint of the Gastroenterologist. Journal of Biological Regulators and Homeostatic Agents. 2018 Apr 26;**32**(4). [Epub ahead of print]

[55] Bianchetti M, Peralta S, Nicita R, Aragona SE, Ciprandi G. The EMERGE (emerging from Gastroesophageal Reflux): an Italian survey—II. The viewpoint of the patient. Journal of Biological Regulators and Homeostatic Agents. 2018 Apr 26;**32**(4). [Epub ahead of print]

[56] Bianchetti M, Peralta S, Nicita R, Aragona SE, Ciprandi G. Correlation between the Reflux Finding Score and the GERD Impact Scale in patients with Gastroesophageal Reflux Disease. Journal of Biological Regulators and Homeostatic Agents. 2018 Apr 26;**32**(4). [Epub ahead of print]

Chapter 5

The Role of Esophagus in Voice Rehabilitation of Laryngectomees

Ljiljana Širić, Marinela Rosso and Aleksandar Včev

Additional information is available at the end of the chapter

http://dx.doi.org/10.5772/intechopen.78594

Abstract

The total laryngectomy is a standard procedure of laryngeal carcinoma treatment which leaves multiple persistent consequences on a laryngectomized person. After laryngectomy, all of patients cannot speak loudly, and 10–58% patients have a dysphagia. In such changed anatomical condition, the esophagus has a key function in two of three primary approaches to voice—speech rehabilitation of laryngectomized patients: esophageal and tracheoesophageal speech therapy method because one of these is the only acceptable solution of substitute alaryngeal speech. In esophageal speech, the esophagus has the role of speech air reservoirs since the respiratory and digestive pathways are permanently separated after the procedure. In the production of tracheoesophageal speech, the tracheoesophageal fistula and the esophagus allow the recommunication of these pathways and the use of air from the lungs for speech. There are several prerequisites for successful esophageal and tracheoesophageal speech. After tracheoesophageal puncture and insertion, the tracheoesophageal prosthesis may occur different complications in the early or late postoperative period in 10–60% of patients. The quality of alaryngeal voice is very different from the quality of laryngeal voice, but allows communication to laryngectomees.

Keywords: esophageal speech, laryngectomy, tracheoesophageal speech, voice prosthesis, voice rehabilitation

1. Introduction

The esophagus is a long, flexible muscular tube that starts as the continuation of the pharynx with the upper esophageal sphincter and ends with the lower esophageal sphincter as the junction with the stomach. Topographically, it is divided into three regions: cervical, thoracic and abdominal [1].

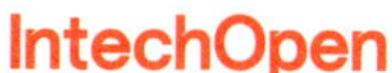

The function of the upper esophageal sphincter is to prevent breathed air from entering into the esophagus and to stop reflux of esophageal content into the pharynx to prevent airway aspiration, and the function of lower esophageal sphincter is to prevent gastroesophageal reflux.

The function of the esophagus is very simple: to actively transport solids and liquids from the pharynx to the stomach. It has no digestive, absorptive, metabolic, or endocrine functions, but in some people, esophagus takes another very important function [2]. These people are laryngectomized persons. Namely, after total laryngectomy, the lower respiratory tract is permanently separated from the upper respiratory tract. The breathing function begins and ends in the permanent tracheostoma, and the upper respiratory tract loses its function [3]. In such anatomical condition, the esophagus has a key function in two of three primary approaches to speech rehabilitation of laryngectomized patients: esophageal and tracheoesophageal speech therapy method. The upper part of the esophagus gets the function as some kind of air activator, and the pharyngoesophageal segment gets the function of the voice generator, thus allowing the function of the voice resonators.

2. Total laryngectomy

The standard options of laryngeal carcinoma treatment are surgery, radiotherapy, chemotherapy, or a combination of these modalities. When a conservation surgery is not indicated due to the tumor stage and localization, or due to patient's general medical condition, then total laryngectomy is considered. This surgical procedure implies a surgical removal of the entire larynx, from the hyoid bone to the second tracheal ring, and the lymph nodes on the ipsilateral or bilateral side. After removal of the larynx, the circular defect in the anterior wall of the pharynx is reconstructed and sutured to the base of the tongue. Inferiorly, resected distal part of trachea is brought forward and sutured to the skin edges forming permanent tracheostoma. Postoperative care after total laryngectomy includes nasogastric tube feedings and maintenance of tracheostoma. If the tracheostoma is satisfactory in size and shape, it is preferable not to use laryngectomy tube in the tracheostoma. Alaryngeal speech training may begin as early as 3 weeks after operation. Postlaryngectomy aphonia is one of the most devastating outcomes of total laryngectomy, and effective voice is critical to the successful prevention of psychological, social and economic consequences of totally laryngectomized individuals [4].

After total laryngectomy, there is a defect of hypopharynx that needs to be reconstructed. The base of tongue then makes anastomosis with neopharynx. Sometimes there is a retraction of the base of tongue, changed tonus of the pharyngoesophageal segment, an extension of a part of pharynx and esophageal stenosis, which can cause dysphagia in 10–58% of cases [5]. Reconstruction of the upper esophageal segment and the hypopharynx is essential for the swallowing function and alaryngeal phonation. In addition, radiotherapy and postoperative infection increases the risk of occurrence of scarring and stenosis of the oropharyngeal segment, causing dysphagia and odynophagia. Postoperative radiotherapy causes other problems such as reduced sense of taste, xerostomia, muscle fibrosis and tooth loss, which increases dysphagic disorders. Therefore, laryngectomees often need to modify their way of nutrition [6].

2.1. Voice rehabilitation after laryngectomy

Total laryngectomy leaves a number of significant and permanent anatomic and physiological-functional changes. One of them is the impossibility of loud laryngeal speech. Laryngectomy is the removal of vocal cords which are the vibrating source of sound, and it causes changes in the anatomic structures of the resonator, whereas tracheotomy prevents the use of the lungs as a physiological source of energy for the phonation. Patient is temporarily socially deprived which diminishes the quality of life and brings with it the limitations in other life spheres. Postoperatively, achieved by rehabilitation, a future alaryngeal voice will be created in the area where esophagus transitions into hypopharynx, under the influence of the airflow that causes the mucosa vibration [5]. This area is called neoglottis or pseudoglottis, and it is a pharyngoesophageal segment, anatomical structure in the area of the upper aerodigestive tract [7].

Rehabilitation of voice after removal of larynx has been known for more than 150 years [8]. The first well-known description of the possible way of producing alaryngeal voice was given by Czermak in 1859. He established an alaryngeal voice by redirecting the airflow from the endotracheal tube through a tube into the mouth of the laryngectomized patient [9]. After Billroth performed his first laryngectomy in 1873, his assistant, Gussenbauer, equipped the patient with a pneumatic device which had the function of a speech machine [8, 10, 11]. In the mid-nineteenth century, rehabilitation was discovered by establishing an esophageal voice. At the same time, various mechanical devices were used to transmit vibrations and thus allowed loud speech [12, 13]. In the mid-twentieth century, the first tracheoesophageal fistula was made, which allowed the air stream to reach the upper part of the esophagus and the pharynx [14]. A few years later, a voice prothesis was developed according to the principle of a one-way permeable valve that allows the airflow from the trachea into the esophagus and prevents the passage of food and fluid from the esophagus into the trachea.

Back a few decades, the world trend is the earliest possible rehabilitation of voice and speech after laryngectomy. The beginning and type of rehabilitation depend on the health, psychosocial and socioeconomic status of the patient [15].

Patients have three methods of substitute voice and speech:

1. Production of tracheoesophageal voice by insertion of a tracheoesophageal prosthesis.
2. Production of an esophageal voice.
3. Use of mechanical generators of acoustic vibrations [16].

3. Esophagus and esophageal speech

3.1. History of the esophageal speech

The use of esophagus as a speech tank for the purpose of rehabilitation of laryngectomized persons first occurs during the nineteenth century. In 1909, Gutzmann called this rehabilitation method an esophageal speech [17]. The method is the most natural way for the laryngectomized persons to have the alaryngeal phonation, which has made it the most commonly used method for many years. Although satisfying a number of factors is a prerequisite, Seeman considers the appropriate level of motivation to be the key factor for mastering the esophageal speech, and that most motivated patients successfully adopt this mode of substitution [17].

3.2. Prerequisites for successful esophageal speech

This method creates a new air reservoir used for speech within the esophagus of a lower capacity than the physiological one, which is the source of the sound wave. The capacity of the upper part of the esophagus after surgery is 60–80 ml of air [18], and the sound wave is generated by vibrations of the pharyngoesophageal segment in neoglottis, which allows the production of the esophageal voice. The exact localization of the pharyngoesophageal segment vibrations differs from author to author, and vibrations are possible from the base of the tongue to the upper esophageal sphincter, but most authors suggest that the most common vibrations of the pharyngoesophageal cavity vibration are at the level of the fifth, sixth and seventh cervical vertebrae, while Seeman feels that vibrations are at the level of the cricopharyngeal muscle at the height of the fifth cervical vertebra or where the pharyngoesophageal obstruction is the greatest [17].

In order for alaryngeal phonation to be possible (production of speech without the larynx), an appropriate tonus of pharyngoesophageal segment, more precisely the cricopharyngeal muscle, is needed. In determining the degree of tonus available, today there are two evaluation tools:

- Taub's insufflation test.
- Modified Taub's test.

When using Taub's Insufflation Test, the examiner places the nasal catheter into the esophagus, using the Polyzer balloon to insufflate the air to the catheter. If the tonus is appropriate, the patient will be able to phonate, and the test will then record a positive result. The reference limit of the phonation pressure is 22 mmHg, which allows the 10 s alaryngeal phonation, or speech production in the range of 10–15 syllables in one inspiration. The phonation pressure is measured with a manometer. In cases where there is hypertonicity, the patient is not able to produce an alaryngeal voice, and the test registers a negative result [19].

The self-blowing test (modified Taube test) has been used for 33 years and was invented by Blom and Singer. The difference is that the other end of the nasal catheter is introduced into the tracheostoma and in this way allows an independent insufflation of the air from the tracheostoma to the esophagus. The result is recorded as positive when the patient can alaryngeally phonate for at least 8 s [20].

The negative result in these tests indicates undesirable hypertonicity of the muscle which prevents the phonation, and requires surgical intervention in the form of cricopharyngeal myotomy [20]. Muscle hypotonicity is also undesirable because it may interfere with alaryngeal phonation, but it often results in a very weak intensity of the alaryngeal voice. As the voice of low intensity does not meet the daily communication requirements, the hypotonicity can be compensated by external compression or surgical intervention.

In addition to the appropriate muscular tonus of the pharyngoesophageal segment, the person who will be rehabilitated with the esophageal speech must have a satisfactory level of certain cognitive abilities. Considered among the most important cognitive abilities are the appropriate intellectual status and the motivation of a person, but the conative factors are also significant. When choosing modality, psychosocial and socioeconomic factors are also important. The person who will learn the esophageal speech should be highly motivated for the process of rehabilitation, be patient enough, cognitively superior, and live in an empathetic and supportive family and social environment. Socioeconomic status should be as high as necessary for regular attendance at a speech-language therapy in continuity. Regarding the health status, people who will learn the esophageal speech should be of a good general health and somatic status, and the primary disease should be under good local control, which means removing any suspicion of local recurrence. Certainly, a significant influence on the possibility of this modality has the auditory status of the patient, and the level of hearing should be appropriate to the chronological age of the person, at the hearing level of 20–55 dB [5]. Any hearing impairment above 55 dB affects the communication function significantly and disables the adequate reception of the information from the speech-language therapist, thereby making it difficult and slowing down the process of rehabilitation.

Doyle classified contraindications for the learning of the esophageal speech in four categories [17, 21, 22]:

1. Certain physical factors
   - local recurrence of illness.
   - extensive reconstruction operation.
2. Certain psychological status
   - the presence of psychological problems and psychopathology.
3. Socioeconomic factors
   - inability to attend a therapy at least three times a week.
4. The necessity of speaking
   - immediately after laryngectomy, the necessity to speak loudly for a certain reason.

3.3. Functional features of the esophageal speech

The acoustic parameters of the esophageal voice in the literature vary depending on the researchers, the selected research method, the measuring instrument, the measuring criteria, the sample of subjects, and the environmental and computer program conditions in which the measurement was performed. The fundamental frequency, or the height of the esophageal voice, is reduced, the frequency range is reduced, and the acoustic parameters determining the timbre of the voice also differ significantly from the regular laryngeal voice [5, 23, 24]. Such values of acoustic parameters form a rough and breathy voice, subjectively experienced. In addition, the time for turning on the voice is prolonged and the maximum time of the phoning is significantly reduced. According to prosodic features, the melody of the esophageal voice is more uniform and variable, lexical stress is not realized or is partially realized, frequent undesirable respiratory pauses are often present and the tempo of speaking is slower [5].

Sociofunctional features of the esophageal voice, which also make the advantage of this rehabilitation modality are: both hands free during speech and being less noticeable to the environment during speech, spontaneous and natural way of alaryngeal speech without additional surgery and insertion of foreign bodies, independence of prosthetic aids, the ability to speak without high consumption of material resources. On the other hand, the features that make up its shortcomings are: long periods of rehabilitation, lack of regular and continuous attendance at rehabilitation, discontinuous speech and additional undesirable noise during speech, especially tracheal noise during inspiration, which interfere with the intelligibility of the pronounced words [25].

3.4. Rehabilitation: educational process of learning the esophageal speech

The rehabilitation and education process starts with an individual preoperative counseling and patient preparation for a postoperative rehabilitation. A duration of the preoperative patient preparation varies depending on the individual's needs. During this period, the patient is given education on all the consequences of tracheotomy and total laryngectomy, pulmonary and speech aids for laryngectomized persons and modalities of speech-language rehabilitation. In addition, an oncological team of experts together with the patient decides on a single rehabilitation method.

The onset of postoperative speech-language therapy depends on a number of factors, such as further oncological treatment (primarily the need for radiotherapy), general health condition, psychological condition, and neuromotor capabilities of the patient. The optimal time to start postoperative rehabilitation is considered 40 days (approximately 6 weeks after surgery) unless postoperative radiotherapy is indicated [26]. However, Remacle and Demard state that rehabilitation can be started earlier, immediately after cicatrization, usually 3 weeks after the operation [17]. If postoperative radiotherapy is indicated, rehabilitation is delayed as long as acute consequences of radiation that hamper the process of rehabilitation are present. Of course, rehabilitation should begin within 6 months of surgery [26]. The total duration of rehabilitation is different and individual.

Early postoperative rehabilitation phase lasts 1 month from the onset of therapy, and primary focus of the therapy is on relaxation techniques and respiratory - rehabilitation operators in physiological breathing onto a tracheostoma to avoid, initially always present, tracheal noise at later phonation.

At this stage, the patient is also educated on how to achieve a ructus. Achieving a ructus is taught by two basic principles in one of three available methods. The first principle is based on the correct technique of injecting speech air into the esophagus, and the other is based on the proper technique of eructation of speech air. **Figure 1** shows the scheme of esophageal voice production.

There are several different methods of introducing speech air into the esophagus used in clinical speech therapy, namely: deglutition, inhalation, injection, blocking, Portman's, Tartapan's, and their combinations [5, 17, 22].

In 1900, Gottstein created and described the deglutition/swallowing method, and Gutzmann supplemented and propagated it. The method requires inserting the required air for the alaryngeal phonation according to the principle of swallowing or air ingestion as a bolus which causes eructation. This is considered the initial method because it allows a volitional ructus, but it affects the rhythm of speech and substantially slows it down, which is its disadvantage. As air swallowing, that is, "dry swallowing" is limited, it is recommended to consume the fluid during therapy [17].

In 1922, Seeman described the inhalation method, also referred to as aspirational or suctioning method. It requires a few swift inhalations that cause a sudden drop in intraoral pressure, which allows aspiration of air from the oral cavity into pharynx, and into the esophagus and relaxation of the pharyngoesophageal segment. When the pressures get equal, the air suction is stopped, the aspirated air is eructated and sounded through the pharyngoesophageal segment. Initially, the vocals are articulated, followed by the syllables made of a combination of gutural/h/ and vocals. Sometimes, the use of the method is followed by hyperventilation. There are several modifications of this method in the world.

The injectable or occlusive method was formed by collecting the experiences of patients who noticed that the easiest way for them to loudly articulate occlusives and syllables combined from occlusives and vocals is alaryngeally. The method requires sufficient pressure of the tongue which causes air compression in the oral cavity and pharynx and is injected into the

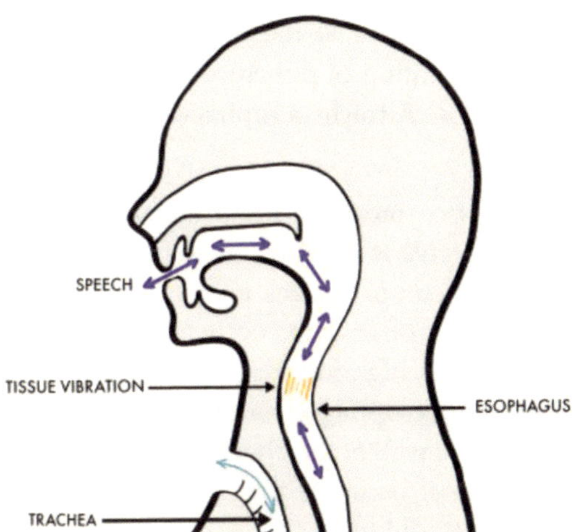

Figure 1. Esophageal voice production.

esophagus, and in the articulation of the labial, alveolar and guttural occlusive the air is liberated and affects the achievement of a satisfactory tonus of the pharyngoesophageal segment. In 1966, Diedrich and Youngstrom created a variation of this method by introducing certain modifications [17].

The blocking method was accomplished by performing several procedures of injectable method followed by specific articulator's movements and by changing the head position. The method involves injecting air from the oral cavity to the esophagus by lip occlusion causing anterior blockage with simultaneous posterior repositioning of the base of the tongue and inferior mandibular repositioning.

By combining several specific procedures from the deglutition and inhalation method, a new method was created by Portman, and was named after him as Portman's method. It requires a few fast-paced air inspirations that are followed by "edacious" deglutition of the air bolus to make speech air flow into the esophagus [22].

In addition, there is Tartapan's method, which is seldom used in clinical speech therapy practice, as well as other possible combinations of existing standard methods that are not specifically described.

4. Esophagus and tracheoesophageal speech

4.1. Tracheoesophageal puncture and tracheoesophageal prosthesis placement

Tracheoesophageal puncture is a surgical method of voice restoration after total laryngectomy that implies creation of a fistulous tract in tracheoesophageal wall—the wall that separates the trachea and esophagus, in the level of tracheostomy. This surgically created fistula which may be formed at the time of the total laryngectomy (primary tracheoesophageal puncture) or after the laryngectomized person has healed from surgery (secondary tracheoesophageal puncture). For satisfactory performance of the tracheoesophageal puncture, an adequate tracheostoma is preferable. The location of puncture is positioned in the midline, 5–10 mm below the mucocutaneous junction. A tracheoesophageal prosthesis is inserted into a fistula, as shown in **Figure 2** [4].

The prosthesis is an artificial device, mostly made of silicone. The purpose of the prosthesis, which is practically "one-way" valve is to allow air to be delivered from the lungs into the esophagus (**Figure 3**). At the same time, the leak of saliva and food in trachea is undesirable and prevented [27]. For this passage of air, good occlusion of the tracheostoma during phonation is necessary. During phonation, high intrathoracic pressure forces the valve to open and directs the air into the upper part of esophagus. Passing of this air into the pharynx and mouth produces vibrations in the mucosal wall of the pharyngoesophageal segment which generates sound. Resonation of the sound occurs in the pharynx, mouth and nose, with simultaneous articulation using the tongue, lips, and teeth.

The most important anatomical part responsible for alaryngeal voice formation is pharyngoesophageal segment. The vibrating pharyngoesophageal segment is the source of sound production and performs vocal cord function. The state of pharyngoesophageal segment made

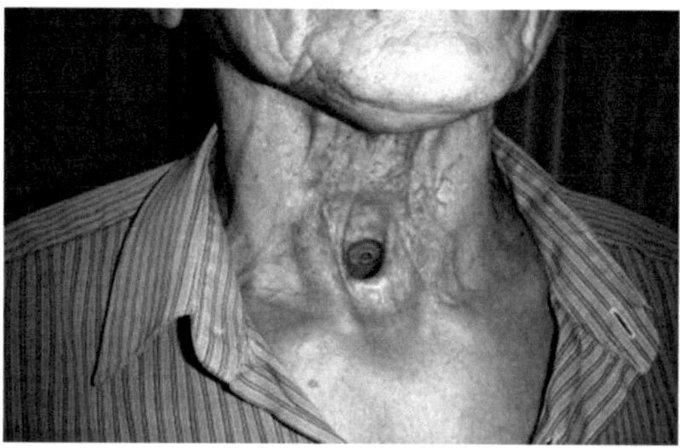

Figure 2. Tracheoesophageal fistula with inserted prosthesis.

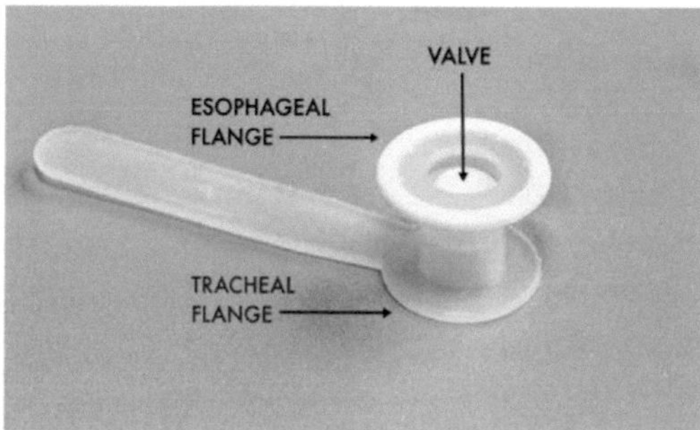

Figure 3. Tracheoesophageal prosthesis.

by the mucosa and surrounding fibers of the repaired cricopharyngeal, thyropharyngeal and the upper esophageal sphincter muscles is very important in voice production, and because of that it is important to preserve as much pharyngeal mucosa as possible at the time of laryngeal surgery [28]. Sometimes PE segment may be hypertonic, spastic or hypotonic. In case that hypertonicity or spasticity is a problem, cricopharyngeal myotomy, pharyngeal neurectomy, PES dilatation or botulinum toxin injection may be beneficial [29].

4.2. History of tracheoesophageal speech

The first experimental prostheses appeared in the second half of the last century, but due to initial structural defects, they could not be cleansed in detail from the secretion, resulting in an infection of the trachea and esophagus [30]. The first silicone tracheoesophageal prosthesis for commercial use was constructed in 1979 and its creators were Blom and Singer [31]. Due to its specific appearance, the prototype of the prosthesis was named duckbill. At the rounded esophageal end, an opening was located with the aim of one-way airflow from the trachea to the esophagus, and at the tracheal end, there was a rim with the extension and the possibility of sticking to the skin to prevent prosthesis from falling out. The second prototype of the prosthesis was created by introducing a one-way valve with a hinged door shape and reduced air resistance. The prostheses were built in secondarily, anterogradely through tracheostoma under general anesthesia. After this, other types of prostheses are created and developed, such as Hermann's prosthesis, Henley-Cohn's prosthesis, Staffieri's prosthesis, Traissac's prosthesis,

Nijdam's prosthesis, Ultra Voice prosthesis, Algaba prosthesis, and Provox prostheses [22]. The primary goal of the prosthesis development was to improve its structural and construction properties with the aim of achieving proper, safe and reliable use, adequate fixation of prosthesis within tracheoesophageal fistula, better prosthesis functionality in terms of low air resistance and greater resistance to fungal and bacterial infections. To date, different manufacturers' tracheoesophageal prostheses of perfected construction and design are available.

4.3. Prerequisites for successful tracheoesophageal voice and speech

The basic requirement for tracheoesophageal prosthesis is the absence of distant metastases or local recurrence [22]. The ability to produce tracheoesophageal voice implies the formation of tracheoesophageal fistula and the insertion of the prosthesis within the tracheoesophageal fistula, which is the surgical method of voice rehabilitation [5].

Andrews, according to Kazi, provides the following indicative criteria of patient's status for inserting the tracheoesophageal prosthesis: motivation, mental stability, sufficient level of comprehension and understanding of the changes in anatomy and functional mechanism of prosthesis and its use, appropriate manual and motor skills, the adequate vision status necessary for the maintenance of the prosthesis, the adequate tonus of hypopharynx, i.e., the absence of stenosis of the hypopharynx, the positive insufflation Taub's test, the tracheostoma of a neat appearance, i.e., the appropriate shape (minimum diameter of 15 mm) and depth, and sufficient lung capacity [32].

4.4. Functional characteristics of tracheoesophageal speech

The tracheoesophageal fistula allows communication between the trachea and esophagus, which is important for the speech because the patient uses the lungs as the air reservoir required for the phonation, which makes the speech more fluent [33], of more appropriate melody and pace with better achieved stresses and fewer respiratory pauses. Although, by acoustic measurements, the fundamental frequency is lowered, and the values of the parameters that determine the timbre are elevated, unlike the esophageal voice, the intensity or volume is greater, and the maximum time of the phonation is longer [5, 24]. If a tracheostoma is occluded manually, patient's hand will be occupied, but this is not necessary because an automatic speech valve can be used for occlusion. The advantage of this method is the duration of rehabilitation, which is considerably shorter than the esophageal speech learning process. The greatest disadvantages of the method are the need to replace prosthesis over a certain period of time and the possibility of developing various speech prosthesis complications or tracheoesophageal fistulas. The average life of the prosthesis is 3–6 months [34].

4.5. Rehabilitation: educational process of learning the tracheoesophageal speech

The rehabilitation process varies depending on the type of prosthesis insertion, whether it is primary, primary postponed or secondary, but the overall process lasts shorter than the esophageal speech learning process. During the tracheoesophageal voice production, it is necessary to occlude the tracheostoma. At the beginning of the rehabilitation, the tracheostoma is occluded with a non-dominant hand, usually by a thumb, to achieve the best occlusion. The complete occlusion of tracheostoma allows the air from the lungs to be directed through the

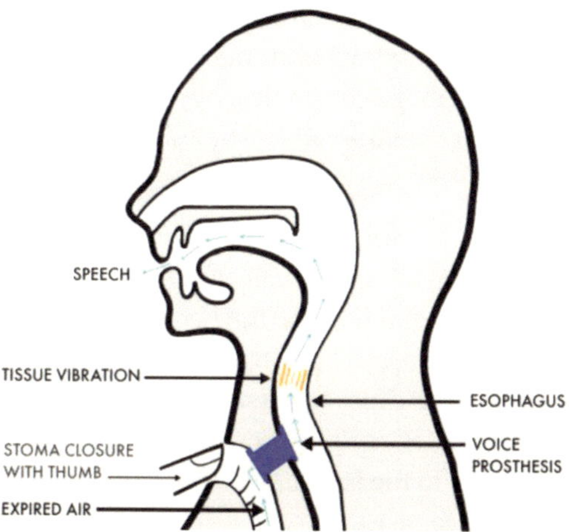

Figure 4. Tracheoesophageal voice production.

trachea and the esophagus into the oral cavity, thereby creating vibration of the pharyngo-esophageal segment and the production of tracheoesophageal speech, while simultaneously preventing undesirable tracheal noise. Rehabilitation begins with rehabilitation-methodical operators of relaxation of the whole body, especially the neck and head, and operators of proper, relaxed, alaryngeal phonation. Once a satisfactory tracheoesophageal phonation is established, the production of this voice articulates the syllables in a combination of silent guttural occlusive and a vocal and then all other sounds. When the patient successfully uses tracheoesophageal voice and speech on a daily basis as the only mean of communication, attention is paid to the details. In order to fix the lack of a free hand, an automatic speech valve is used. The automatic speech valve consists of a plastic casing inside which is located the membrane for controlling the flow of the economical amount of air and the filter for maintaining the temperature and humidity of the air [34].

Rehabilitation ends when a patient can produce spontaneous speech without significant difficulties, that is, when tracheostoma is well-occluded, a voice of satisfactory quality, speech is intelligible, and when the patient uses tracheoesophageal speech as the main mean of communication. **Figure 4** shows the scheme of tracheoesophageal voice production.

The assessment of the performance of voice-speech rehabilitation is performed using the Harrison and Robillard-Schultz scales for assessing tracheoesophageal voice and speech, including a sub-scale for assessing the maintenance of tracheoesophageal prosthesis [35].

4.6. Tracheoesophageal puncture and tracheoesophageal prosthesis complications

Complications may occur in the early or late postoperative period in 10–60% of patients [34, 36, 37] and may be divided into:

1. Complications of tracheoesophageal puncture.
2. Complications of tracheoesophageal fistula.
3. Complications of tracheoesophageal prosthesis.

Complications of tracheoesophageal puncture are complications resulting from the surgical procedure itself, and among them are tracheostoma of inadequate form, size and depth, inadequate tonus of the pharyngoesophageal segment (hypotonicity or hypertonicity) [38] and the formation of pseudoepiglottis or pseudo-vallecula [39].

Complications of tracheoesophageal fistula occur in later postoperative period, most commonly the same patient having several different complications. Among these complications are the atrophy of the tracheoesophageal wall, tracheal mucosa granulation, esophageal mucosa hypertrophy, increase in diameter of tracheoesophageal fistulae, dislocation of the voice prosthesis and leakage of the esophagus from the voice prosthesis into the trachea [40]. Inadequate size of voice prosthesis causes pressure on the esophageal and tracheal mucosa and may result in fibromatous reactions [39]. Several cases of decubitus of the back esophageal wall have been reported due to the incompatibility of the length of the tracheoesophageal fistula with the length of the voice prosthesis.

The complications of the tracheoesophageal prosthesis are the release of one-way prosthesis valves, resulting in leakage of the esophagus through the voice prosthesis into the trachea [41, 42], and the creation of biofilm in the voice prosthesis due to its use during several months [43, 44].

5. Conclusion

The physiological function of the esophagus in healthy people is very simple: to actively transport solids and liquids from the pharynx to the stomach. It has no digestive, absorptive, metabolic, or endocrine functions, but in laryngectomized persons, esophagus takes one more function. In such changed anatomical condition, the esophagus has a key role in voice—speech rehabilitation of laryngectomized patients because the esophageal and tracheoesophageal speech are the only acceptable solution of substitute alaryngeal speech. The esophagus gets very important function at alaryngeal phonation as air reservoir, the upper esophageal sphincter gets the function as air activator and the pharyngoesophageal segment gets the function of the voice generator, thus allowing the function of the voice resonators.

Acknowledgements

We would like to thank Ms. Mirna Brunčić for translating this text.

Notes

The figures are from the author's own source.

Conflict of interest

The authors have no conflict of interest.

Author details

Ljiljana Širić[1]*, Marinela Rosso[2] and Aleksandar Včev[3]

*Address all correspondence to: ljsiric@gmail.com

1 Department of Otorhinolaryngology and Head and Neck Surgery, University Hospital Centre Osijek, Osijek, Croatia

2 Polyclinic Rosso, Osijek, Croatia

3 Faculty of Medicine, J. J. Strossmayer University of Osijek, Osijek, Croatia

References

[1] Sabiston DC, Sellke FW, Del NPJ, Swanson SJ. Sabiston & Spencer Surgery of the Chest. Philadelphia: Saunders/Elsevier; 2010

[2] Rice TW. Esophagus. In: Norton JA et al, editors. Surgery. Berlin, Heidelberg: Springer; 2001

[3] Hilgers FJM, Ackerstaff AH. Comprehensive rehabilitation after total laryngectomy is more than voice alone. Folia Phoniatrica et Logopaedica. 2000;**52**:65-73

[4] Shah JP, Patel SG. Head and Neck Surgery and Oncology. Edinburgh: Mosby; 2003

[5] Širić Lj. Utjecaj vrste alaringealne fonacije na akustičke parametre glasa i prozodijske elemente govora. [Doktorska disertacija]. Osijek: Sveučilište J. J. Strossmayera Osijek, Medicinski fakultet; 2017

[6] Rosso M. Utjecaj kazeta za održavanje vlažnosti i temperature zraka na morfološki i funkcionalni status donjih dišnih putova laringektomiranih osoba. [Doktorska disertacija]. Osijek: Sveučilište J. J. Strossmayera Osijek, Medicinski fakultet; 2015

[7] Van der Torn M. A sound-producing voice prosthesis [Doctoral dissertation]. Amsterdam: Vrije University Medical Center; 2005

[8] Hirokazu S, Takahashi H. Voice generation system using an intra-mouth vibrator for the laryngectomee [Master's thesis]. Japan: University of Tokyo; 2000

[9] Czermak J. Uber die Sprache bei luftdichter Verschliessung des Kehlkopfs. Wien: Sitzungsberichte der kaiserlichen Academie der Wissenschafter mathematischnaturwissenschaftliche Classe; 1859

[10] Gussenbauer C. Ueber die erste durch Th. Billroth am Menschen ausgefuerte Kehlkopf – Extirpation und die Anwendung eines Kuenstlichen Kehlkopfes. Archiv Fur Klinische Chirurgie. 1874;**17**:343-356

[11] Weir N. Otolaryngology: An Illustrated History London: Butterworths; 1990

[12] Struebbing PDL. Pseudostimme nach Ausschaltung des Kehlkopfs, speziell nach Extirpation desselben. Deutsche Medizinische Wochenschrift. 1988;**14**:1061

[13] Struebbing PDL. Erzeugung einer (natuerlichen) Pseudo – Stimme bei einem Manne mit totaler Extirpation des Kehlkopfes. Archiv Fur Klinische Chirurgie. 1889;**38**:142

[14] Lowry LD. Artificial larynges: a review and development of a prototype selfcontained intra-oral artificial larynx. Laryngoscope. 1981;**91**(8):1332-1355

[15] Fagan JJ, Lentin R, Oyarzabal MF, Isaacs S, Sellars SL. Tracheoesophageal speech in a developing worldcommunity. Archives of Otolaryngology – Head & Neck Surgery. 2002;**128**(1):50-53

[16] Brown DH, Hilgers FJM, Irish JC, Balm AJ. Postlaryngectomy voice rehabilitation: State of the art at the millennium. World Journal of Surgery. 2003;**27**(7):824-831

[17] Stanković DP. Fonijatrijska rehabilitacija laringtomisanih pacijenata uspostavljanjem ezofagusnog glasa i govora modificiranom Semanovom metodom [Doktorska disertacija]. Beograd: Univerzitet u Beogradu, Medicinski fakultet; 1997

[18] Mahieu HF. Voice and speech Rehabilitation following laryngectomy [Doctoral thesis]. Groningen: Rijk University Groningen; 1988

[19] Taub S, Bergner LH. Air bypass voice prosthesis for vocal rehabilitation of laryngectomees. American Journal of Surgery. 1973;**125**:748-756

[20] Blom ED, Singer MI, Hamaker RC. A prospective study of tracheo-oesophageal speech. Archives of Otolaryngology-Head and Neck Surgery. 1986;**112**:440-447

[21] Doyle PC. Foundations of voice and speech Rehabilitation following laryngeal Cancer San Diego: Singular Publishing Group Inc; 1994

[22] Dragičević D. Govorna rehabilitacija totalno laringektomisanih pacijenata ugradnjom vokalnih proteza [Doktorska disertacija]. Medicinski fakultet Novi Sad: Novi Sad; 2013

[23] Milutinović Z. Studija glasa posle lečenja karcinoma larinksa. Nova knjiga: Beograd; 1985

[24] Širić LJ, Šoš D, Rosso M, Stevanović S. Objective assessment of tracheoesophageal and esophageal voice using acoustic analysis of voice. Collegium Antropologicum 2012;**36**: 111-114

[25] Štajner-Katušić S. Glas i govor nakon totalne laringektomije. Grafostil: Zagreb; 1998

[26] Mumović GM. Konzervativni tretman disfonija. Medicinski fakultet Novi Sad: Novi Sad; 2004

[27] Blom ED, Hamaker RC. Tracheoesophageal voice restoration following total laryngectomy. In: Myers EN, Suen J, editors. Cancer of the Head and Neck. 3rd ed. Philadelphia: W.B. Saunders Company; 1996. pp. 839-852

[28] Kotby MN, Hegazi MA, Kamal I, Gamal El Dien N, Nassar J. Aerodynamics of the pseudo-glottis. Folia Phoniatrica et Logopaedica. 2009;**61**:24-28

[29] Arenaz B, Rydell R, Westin U, Olsson R. The pharyngoesophageal segment in laryngectomees with non-functional voice: Is it all about spasm? Journal of Otology & Rhinology. 2016;**5**:4. DOI: 10.4172/2324-8785.1000287

[30] Hilgers FJM, Ackerstaff AH, Balm AJ, et al. Development and clinical evaluation of a second-generation voice prosthesis (Provox 2), designed for anterograde and retrograde insertion. Acta Oto-Laryngologica. 1997;**117**(6):889-896

[31] Singer MI, Blom ED. An endoscopic technique for restoration of voice after laryngectomy. Annals of Otology. 1980;**89**:529-533

[32] Andrews JC, Mickel RA, Hanson DG, Monahan GP. Major complications following tracheoesophageal puncture for voice rehabilitation. The Laryngoscope. 1987;**97**:562-567

[33] Lorenz KJ, Groll K, Ackerstaff AH, Hilgers FJM, Maier H. Hands-free speech after surgical voice rehabilitation with a Provox voice prosthesis: Experience with the Provox free hands HME tracheostoma valve system. European Archives of Oto-Rhino-Laryngology. 2006;**264**(2):151-157

[34] Capaccio P, Schnidler A, Tassone G, Ottaviani F. Comparative study of esophageal and tracheo-esophageal voice by digital spectrographic analysis. Acta Phoniatrica Latina. 2001;**23**:322-326

[35] Op de Coul B, Hilgers F, Balm A, Tan I, van den Hoogen F, Van Tinteren H. A decade of postlaryngectomy vocal rehabilitation in 318 patients: A single institutions experience with consistent application of provox indwelling voice prostheses. Archives of Otolaryngology – Head & Neck Surgery 2000;**126**:1320-1328

[36] Lukinović J, Bilić M, Raguž I, Živković T, Kovač-Bilić L, Prgomet D. Overview of 100 patients with voice prosthesis after total laryngectomy-Experience of single institution. Collegium Antropologicum. 2012;**36**:99-102

[37] Malik T, Bruce I, Cherry J. Surgical complications of tracheo-oesophageal puncture and speech valves. Current Opinion in Otolaryngology & Head and Neck Surgery. 2007;**15**:117-122

[38] Brok H, Stroeve R, Copper M, Schouwenburg P. The treatment of hypertonicity of the pharyngo-oesophageal segment after laryngectomy. Clinical Otolaryngology. 1998;**23**: 302-307

[39] Đanić Hadžibegović A. Utjecaj ekstraezofagealnog refluksa na učestalost komplikacija i kvalitetu glasa bolesnika s govornom protezom [Doktorska disertacija]. Zagreb: Sveučilište u Zagrebu, Medicinski fakultet; 2013

[40] Balm AJM, Van den Brekel MWM, Tan IB, Hilgers FJM. The indwelling voice prosthesis for speech rehabilitation after total laryngectomy: A safe approach. Otolaryngologia Polska. 2011;**65**:402-409

[41] Soolsma J, Van den Brekel M, Ackerstaff A, Balm A, Tan I, Hilgers F. Long-term results of Provox ActiValve, solving the problem of frequent Candida and "Underpressure"-related voice prosthesis replacements. Laryngoscope. 2008;**118**:252-257

[42] Leder SB, Acton LM, Kmiecik J, Ganz C, Blom ED. Voice restoration with the advantage tracheoesophageal voice prosthesis. Otolaryngology and Head and Neck Surgery. 2005;**133**:681-684

[43] Smith A, Buchinsky FJ, Post JC. Eradicating chronic ear, nose and throat infections. Otolaryngology and Head and Neck Surgery. 2011;**144**:338-347

[44] Mahieu H, Van Saene J, Den Besten J, Van Saene H. Oropharynx decontamination preventing Candida vegetations on voice prostheses. Archives of Otolaryngology – Head & Neck Surgery. 1986;**112**:1090-1092